Stress and Health

Stress and Health

For Consumers, Healthcare Providers, Patients and Physicians

Eugene A. DeFelice, M.D., F.A.P.M.

iUniverse, Inc.
New York Lincoln Shanghai

Stress and Health
For Consumers, Healthcare Providers, Patients and Physicians

iUniverse books may be ordered through booksellers or by contacting:

iUniverse
2021 Pine Lake Road, Suite 100
Lincoln, NE 68512
www.iuniverse.com
1-800-Authors (1-800-288-4677)

The information, ideas and suggestions in this book are not intended as a substitute for professional medical advice. Before following any suggestions contained in this book, you should first consult your personal physician. Neither the author nor the publisher shall be liable or responsible for any loss or damage allegedly arising as a consequence of your use or application of any information or suggestions in this book.

ISBN-13: 978-0-595-41065-1 (pbk)
ISBN-13: 978-0-595-85426-4 (ebk)
ISBN-10: 0-595-41065-0 (pbk)
ISBN-10: 0-595-85426-5 (ebk)

Printed in the United States of America

This book is dedicated to Ms. Maryanne Harvey, M.S., who has devoted her professional career to the betterment of the health and welfare of others as a member of management the New York State Department of Health. Maryanne's very able professional advice and assistance served to make publication of this book possible.

Acknowledgements

The author acknowledges that the Web Resources/Websites in the Author's List, and additional ones cited in the text, provided the information presented in this book and are hereby credited accordingly.

Contents

Acknowledgements vii

Preface xv

Chapter 1—The Stress Response 1

    1.1   What is Stress 1

    1.2   Overall Response to Stress 3

    1.3   Brain's Response to Stress 3

    1.4   Heart, Lungs and Circulation Response to Stress 4

    1.5   Immune System Response to Stress 4

    1.6   Skin's Response to Stress 5

    1.7   Metabolic Response to Stress 5

    1.8   Good and Bad Stress 5

    1.9   Stress Overload 6

    1.10 Health Consequences of Stress 8

    1.11 Relaxation Response: Resolution of Stress 16

Chapter 2—Stress Risk Factors 17

    2.1   Abusive Behavior 17

    2.2   Angry Personalities 18

    2.3   Caregiving 18

    2.4   City Dwelling 19

2.5	Chronic Exposure to Stress	19
2.6	Divorced or Widowed	19
2.7	Genetic Factors	19
2.8	Immune Disorders	19
2.9	Isolation	19
2.10	Mothers Who Work	20
2.11	Racial or Sexual Discrimination	20
2.12	Relaxation Response Failure	20
2.13	Social Network Deficiency	20
2.14	Uneducated, Unemployed, Uninsured	21
2.15	Work	21
2.16	Worries, Real or Imagined	22

Chapter 3—Happiness, Unhappiness and Stress **23**

3.1	Purpose of Life	23
3.2	Happiness and Unhappiness	24
3.3	Happiness—Research Findings	26
3.4	Love	29
3.5	Pursuit of Happiness	31
3.6	Psychiatrists, Physicians and Antidepressants Do Not Cure Unhappiness	32
3.7	Gratitude, Stress Reduction, and Happiness	33
3.8	Five Roads to Happiness	35

Chapter 4—Anger and Stress **42**

4.1	What is Anger	42
4.2	Aggressive Driving	44
4.3	Domestic violence	45
4.4	Intermittent Explosive Disorder (IED)	45

4.5   Self Assessment: Just How Angry Are You? 46

4.6   Anger: Effect on Health 47

4.7   Anger Management 49

Chapter 5—Caregiving Stress 52

5.1   Caregiving 52

5.2   Caregiving Stress 54

5.3   Caregiving and Controlling Frustration 55

5.4   Prevention and Controlling Caregiving Stress 56

5.5   Elder Abuse and Neglect 57

5.6   Relieving Caregiving Stress 58

5.7   Respite Care 59

5.8   National Family Caregiver Support Program (NFCSP) 60

5.9   Caregiving Resources in One's Community 60

Chapter 6—Family Stress 64

6.1   Introduction 64

6.2   Aspects of Family Stress 65

6.3   Family Changes and Stress 67

6.4   Ways to Reduce Family Stress 68

Chapter 7—Financial Stress 73

7.1   Introduction 73

7.2   Warning Signs of Too Much Debt 75

7.3   Budgeting Improves One's Financial Life 76

7.4   Budget Breakers that May Ruin Your Financial Life 76

7.5   Lay the Foundation for Financial Freedom 78

7.6   Help is Available Now for Financial Stress 79

Chapter 8—Job Stress **81**

    8.1   Introduction 81

    8.2   Economic Impact 81

    8.3   Causes of Job Stress 82

    8.4   Job Stress and Health 83

    8.5   Prevention of Job Stress 84

    8.6   Job Burnout 86

    8.7   Job Success 87

Chapter 9—Stress Management Guidelines and Principles **89**

    9.1   Guidelines 89

    9.2   Principles 91

    9.2.1   Prevention 91

    9.2.2   Adopt a Healthy Lifestyle 92

    9.2.3   Strategies for Keeping Stress under Control 93

Chapter 10—Stress Management—Relaxation Techniques **100**

    10.1   Breathing Exercises 100

    10.2   Cognitive Behavior Therapy 101

    10.3   Hypnosis—Self-Hypnosis/Mental Imagery—Visualization 103

    10.4   Massage Therapy 107

    10.5   Meditation 108

    10.6   Progressive Muscle Relaxation 109

    10.7   Tai Chi 110

    10.8   Yoga 111

    10.9   Spirituality, Stress and Health 112

    10.9.1   Centering Prayer 113

    10.9.2   Peace Prayer of St. Francis of Assisi 113

10.9.3   The Author's Prayer 115

10.9.4   Serenity Prayer 115

Chapter 11—Searching the Web **118**

Chapter 12—Author's List: Stress Web Resources/Websites **121**

12.1   About.com/a New York Times Company 121
         http://www.about.com/stress

12.2   American Academy of Family Physicians (AAFP) 122
         http://www.aafp.org

12.3   American College of Preventive Medicine (ACPM) 124
         http://www.acpm.org

12.4   American Institute of Stress (AIS) 126
         http://www.stress.org

12.5   American Psychiatric Association (APA) 128
         http://www.psych.org

12.6   American Psychological Association (APA) 129
         http://www.apa.org

12.7   Family Doctor (FD) 132
         http://www.familydoctor.org

12.8   HealthFinder (HF) 134
         http://www.healthfinder.gov

12.9   Mayo Clinic (MC) 135
         http://www.mayoclinic.com

12.10   MedicineNet (MN) 138
         http://www.medicinenet.com

12.11   MedlinePlus (MP) 139
         http://www.medlineplus.gov

12.12   Mental Help Net (MHN) 141
         http://www.mentalhelp.net

12.13   Mind Body Medical Institute (MBMI) 146
        http://www.mbmi.org

12.14   National Institute for Occupational Safety and Health
        (NIOSH) 147
        http://www.cdc.gov/niosh/homepage.html

12.15   National Institute of Mental Health (NIMH) 150
        http://www.nimh.nih.gov

12.16   National Mental Health Association (NMHA) 151
        http://www.nmha.org

12.17   WebMD 152
        http://www.webmd.com

Chapter 13—About the Author 154

Preface

Most individuals do not lead a healthy lifestyle or devote sufficient attention to their health and wellness. Those who do not lead a healthy lifestyle should consider that:

> First we squander health in search of wealth,
> We work and toil and save.
> Then we squander wealth in search of health,
> And find an early grave.
>
> Anonymous

A healthy lifestyle is essential for good health, happiness, well-being and longevity. An unhealthy one is stressful and often leads to chronic disease, disability, unhappiness, and a shortened life span.

More than fifty percent of Americans say they are concerned with the amount of stress in their lives. As a result, the United States now is recognized as a "stressed out nation".

Many Americans now react to a variety of stresses in their lives by engaging in unhealthy behaviors such as comfort overeating, making poor diet choices, smoking, abusing alcohol and drugs, and leading a sedentary and unhealthy lifestyle.

Stress affects both mind and body health in a variety of ways. According to an American Psychological Association survey, in partnership with the

National Women's Health Resource Center, the leading sources of stress in the United States are reported to be:

- 59%, money
- 59%, work
- 53%, health problems affecting family members
- 50%, personal health concerns
- 50%, nightly news or state of world today
- 41%, children

And, those feeling stressed report the following effects:

- 59%, nervous and/or sad
- 56%, unable to sleep well
- 55%, lack of interest, motivation or energy
- 51%, symptoms of fatigue
- 48%, muscle tension
- 46%, headache
- 37%, changes in appetite
- 32%, frequent upset stomach or indigestion
- 29%, faint or dizzy
- 26%, tightness in chest
- 23%, change in sex drive

Stress and its associated diseases/disorders are now reported to be responsible for a large proportion of disability worldwide and expected to reach over 50% of the population by the year 2020.

The World Health Organization (WHO) Global Burden of Disease Survey estimates that mental disease, including stress-related disorders, will be the second leading cause of disabilities by the year 2020.

The Cleveland Clinic, one of the foremost medical centers, recently spoke to the American stress problem in the Wall Street Journal (Tuesday, July 18, 2006, pA5) highlighting the scope of the problem and the need for treatment for the "overstressed, overworked, over caffeinated Americans everywhere".

Although the term "stress" is used in a wide variety of contexts, it has been consistently demonstrated that individuals with stress and related disorders experience: 1) impaired physical and mental functioning, 2) more work days lost, 3) loss of productivity at work, and 4) high use of health care services.

While it is difficult to know the true dollar amount of the economic cost of stress and stress-related disorders, it is estimated to be in the hundreds of billions of dollars annually in the United States alone. Thus, early recognition of the toll of the stress problem and the allocation of more resources devoted to prevention and management, is expected to provide significant benefits to individuals affected and the nation as well.

References:

- American Psychological Association

  Stressed Out Nation

  http://www.apa.org/monitor/apr06/nation.html

  Americans Engage in Unhealthy Behaviors to Manage Stress

  http://www.apa.org/releases/stresssurvey0206.html

- *Assessing the Economic Impact of Stress—The Modern Day Hidden Epidemic*

  By Kalia, M., 2002

  PubMed ID:12040542

Eugene A. DeFelice, M.D.

2006

Chapter 1 — The Stress Response

1.1   What is Stress

"Stress is the non-specific response of the body to any demand made on it" according to the late and illustrious Hans Selye, MD, a key pioneer in modern medicine and stress research. Stress responses generally include essentially the "entire body"—e.g., the brain, internal organs, the immune, nervous and cardiovascular systems, and skin. Whenever one is called upon to react/adapt to internal or external factors called stressors, one undergoes a stress response. And, this may occur as a result of a wide variety of pleasant or unpleasant events/experiences such as:

- abuse
- anger
- auto accident
- crime victim
- death of a spouse, child, close family member or friend
- disease
- divorce
- family conflict/discord
- harmful event
- job loss
- natural disasters
- pain
- trauma
- worry regarding real or imagined events/experiences

Such common stressors may produce physiological and/or psychological manifestations of stress.

The stress response is the body's automatic reaction to the stress it receives or perceives. It includes the changes necessary to respond and adapt to that stress. Stress is everywhere present and difficult to avoid in the process of everyday living. It enables the body to rise to the occasion and meet the change/challenge at hand with the heightened alertness, focus, strength, and stamina necessary to bring about successful adaptation.

As noted above, events/experiences that provoke stress range from outright physical danger as when being attacked, to making a speech, taking an exam or facing an important job interview.

Stressors may be divided into short-term (acute) or long term (chronic, over 3–6 months in duration).

Short-term or acute stress is the reaction to an immediate threat, commonly known as the fight or flight response. The threat can be any situation that is experienced, either real or imagined, as a danger. Under the vast majority of circumstances, once the acute threat has passed, the stress response is inactivated and levels of stress hormones return to normal, a condition known as the "relaxation response". As a result, acute stress is usually of little consequence to health and well-being.

Chronic stress, on the other hand, concerns the reality that modern life often imposes an extra burden on stressful situations that are not short-lived and the urge to act quickly is suppressed. In such situations, stress may remain present, become chronic, and pose a significant threat to one's physical and/or mental health as a result.

Adaptation or coping remains the key to handling stress. Ways to accomplish this are covered in Chapters 9 and 10 on Stress Management.

The importance of adaptation is described in one of the best definitions of the human mind quoted in the book "The Human Mind" by Karl Meninger, Alfred A. Knoff, 1946:

"All our lives long, every day and every hour, we are engaged in the process of accommodating our changed and unchanged selves to changed and unchanged surroundings.

Living in fact is nothing else than this process of accommodation. When we fail in it a little, we are stupid, when we fail flagrantly we are mad, when we suspend it temporarily we sleep, and when we give up the attempt all together we die. In quiet, uneventful lives, the changes internal and external are so small that there is little or no strain in the process of fusion and accommodation. In other lives, there is great strain, but there also is great fusing and accommodating power; in others great strain with little accommodating power.

A life will be successful or not as the power of accommodation is equal or unequal to the strain of fusing and adjusting internal and external changes".

Samuel Butler, *The Way of All Flesh*, Penguin Books, 1986, p.327

1.2   Overall Response to Stress

In response to stress, a part of the brain known as the hypothalamic-pituitary-adrenal (HPA) axis becomes activated.

The HPA system triggers the production and release of steroid hormones called glucocorticoids from the adrenal glands, including the key stress hormone, cortisol. This hormone is important in marshalling various organ systems throughout the body to adapt to the stress at hand. These body systems marshaled to adapt include the brain, nervous system, heart, lungs, circulation, metabolism, immune system and skin.

1.3   Brain's Response to Stress

The HPA system also releases certain chemical messengers, the catecholamines, particularly dopamine, epinephrine, and norepinephrine which:

- Activate an area inside the brain called the amygdala, believed to trigger an emotional response to a stressful event/experience such as fear.

- Send signals to a nearby area of the brain called the hippocampus which stores emotionally loaded experiences essential for survival into long-term memory, especially when such memory is vital for avoiding such threats in the future.

- Suppress activity in areas at the front of the brain concerned with short-term memory, concentration, inhibition, and rational thought. This sequence of mental events allows one to react quickly, to fight or flee, as the case may demand. However, it also hinders the ability to handle complex social or intellectual tasks and behavior.

1.4   Heart, Lungs and Circulation Response to Stress

The heart, lungs and circulation respond vigorously to stress, namely:

- heart rate and blood pressure increase;

- breathing becomes rapid/lungs take in more oxygen;

- blood flow increases significantly, priming the muscles, lungs, and brain to meet demands;

- spleen discharges red and white blood cells allowing the blood to transport more oxygen, and combat injury.

1.5   Immune System Response to Stress

The immune system responds to stress when steroid hormones stimulate white blood cells and/or immune molecular substances to be released and redistributed optimally to fight trauma and infection.

1.6 Skin's Response to Stress

Fluids are diverted from non-essential areas of the body such as the skin, mouth and throat. This causes dryness of the mouth and difficulty in talking. In addition, stress can cause spasms of the throat muscles, making it difficult to swallow. Blood flow is diverted away from skin to support heart and muscle tissues. The effect may be a cool, clammy, sweaty skin. The scalp also tightens so that the hair may seem to stand-up.

1.7 Metabolic Response to Stress

Stress decreases digestive activity, especially during short-term periods of physical exertion or crisis.

1.8 Good and Bad Stress

There are essentially two main categories of stress, namely:

- Eustress = good, normal, usually positive and pleasant stress
- Distress = bad, abnormal, usually negative and unpleasant stress. This is the stress of concern for well-being and health—"the stress of excess", both in terms of intensity and/or chronic nature, which can interfere with normal every day living activities, productivity, well-being, health, and longevity.

There appears to be a direct relationship between stress and human productivity. With low level stress, human productivity usually is low—as also is the case with high levels of stress. On the other hand, optimal levels of health, longevity and productivity appear to be linked to moderate levels of eustress and the associated normal anxiety/arousal produced. As satisfaction and success in life in our materialistic Western civilization appears to depend in a large measure on productivity and advancement, a moderate amount of eustress seems essential in this sense.

In addition, individuals seek and enjoy a moderate amount of eustress in the form of adventure, excitement, and challenge. Mild to moderate degrees of eustress for short periods of time are of little concern for health and may even be considered helpful in increasing progress in life, well-being and happiness.

The stress response is critical during emergency situations. It also can be activated in a milder form at a time when the pressure is on but there is no actual danger—like hitting a golf ball over a water hazard in an important golf match, meeting someone for the first time in a job interview, or waiting to go on a long awaited vacation trip. Eustress can help keep you on your toes and ready to rise to a challenge. In such cases, the stress response system responds and quickly returns to its normal state, standing by to respond again as needed.

However, stress doesn't always happen in response to stressors that are short-term or over quickly. Longer term events/experiences, like coping with the death of a close friend or family member, a drawn-out contested divorce, moving to a new job, chronic disease/pain, etc., can cause distress. Chronic stressful situations can produce a lasting level of distress that is hard on an individual's health and well-being. In such cases, the mind senses continued pressure, remains activated, and continues to pump out extra stress hormones/catecholamines over an extended period, leaving a person feeling anxious and/or depressed, depleted, overwhelmed, and with a weakened immune system. This can cause one or more health problems or serious mental and/or bodily disorders/disease. The scope of this book is devoted chiefly to this form of stress, namely distress.

1.9   Stress Overload

While a mild to moderate amount of eustress can be a good thing, stress overload especially in the form of distress, is a different story. Distress isn't good for anyone. For example, feeling a little stress about an upcoming vacation/trip can motivate one to plan things to ensure it will be successful and avoid pitfalls. But "stressing-out" too much over the trip can make it difficult to plan successfully or enjoy the experience.

Stress that is too intense, lasts too long, or is shouldered alone, can cause one to feel stress overload. Stressors that may overwhelm the ability of the mind or body to cope may include such things as:

- being physically or psychologically abused;
- "broken heart" or death of a loved one;
- career crisis/loss of job/forced early retirement;
- continuing financial crisis;
- contested divorce;
- crammed schedule;
- exposure to violence or injury;
- handling continuing emotional problems of everyday living;
- mental anguish that can accompany a mid-life or other crisis;
- ongoing problems related to work or education;
- relationship/family conflicts.

Stressful situations can be extreme and may require special attention and care. Post-traumatic stress disorder can develop in individuals who have lived through a traumatic event such as a terrorist attack, war time combat service, a serious car accident, a natural disaster like a flood or an earthquake, or an assault like rape or robbery.

Individuals who suffer from anxiety and/or depression or other mental disorders can overreact to stress, making even small difficulties/stress responses seem like crises.

Those that continually or frequently feel tense, upset, worried or distressed, may be suffering from stress overload and may benefit from professional counseling/therapy from their healthcare provider/physician.

Individuals experiencing stress overload may display signs/symptoms of:

- allergy or asthma
- anger excess
- anxiety
- depression
- drinking too much
- eating disorder
- family discord/conflict
- irritability
- mental illness
- overeating and weight gain/loss
- panic attacks
- sleep problems
- substance abuse

Stress affects individuals differently. Some may become angry and act out their stress or take it out on others—usually those closer to the affected individual. Others may internalize the stress and develop cardiovascular, gastrointestinal, eating disorders, skin afflictions, or mental disorders such as anxiety, depression, panic, or substance abuse. And, some people who already have a chronic illness may find that the symptoms/signs of their illness flare up and worsen under an overload of stress.

1.10   Health Consequences of Stress

Before modern civilization evolved, physical changes in response to stress were essential for meeting natural threats and to ensure survival.

In more modern times, the stress response may be regarded as an asset for raising levels of performance in work and sports activities, or in actual situations of danger or crisis such as a hurricane or a terrorist attack.

However, when stress becomes persistent and chronic over time, organ systems of the body (brain, heart, immune and circulatory systems, lungs, muscles and skin) become chronically activated, and this may produce physical and/or psychological damage to health and well-being.

Even acute stress may be harmful and cause disease and even death under certain circumstances. Numerous studies indicate that the inability to adapt satisfactorily to stress is associated with the onset of anxiety, depression, post-traumatic stress disorder or other mental disorders. Most individuals experiencing a significant stressful situation appear to have increased risk of developing anxiety and/or depression within a month of the event. Evidence indicates that chronic, repeated release of stress hormones may produce hyperactivity of the HPA axis, adversely affecting normal levels of brain serotonin, the neurotransmitter involved in the feeling of well-being. And, stress may diminish not only the overall quality of life and feelings of pleasure and accomplishment, but also may negatively affect relationships.

Some selected health problem examples that may result from stress include:

- **Allergy**

  Stress may actually produce allergies such as asthma, eczema, and sinus problems not only in office workers but also in the home. This appears to be particularly true in dwellings constructed to conserve air and limit cold and heat exchanges.

- **Anxiety**

  While anxiety may manifest a number of the physical symptoms of stress such as increased heart rate, shallow rapid breathing, and increased muscle tension, it is considered to be primarily an emotional disorder characterized by feelings of apprehension, uncertainly, fear, or panic. Triggers for anxiety are not necessarily associated with specific stressful or threatening conditions. Moreover, chronic stress may result in anxiety disorders that may cause increased stress.

- **Cancer**

  Current evidence does not appear to support stress as a cause for cancer in humans. However, some animal studies indicate that lack of control over stress has negative effects on immune function and contributes to tumor growth. In some studies in patients with either breast cancer or melanoma, improved survival has been reported with therapies that provided emotional support. And, support groups are believed to offer value in reducing stress in patients with terminal cancer.

- **Cardiovascular disease**

  Acute and chronic stress are associated with a significantly higher risk for serious cardiac events such as angina (chest pain due to coronary artery disease), arrhythmias (heart rhythm abnormalities), heart attacks, and even death from such events, especially in individuals with underlying cardiovascular disease.

  The release of stress hormone negatively affects the heart and the rest of the cardiovascular system in several ways. Stress:

  - Alters heart rhythm, increasing the risk for serious arrhythmias, especially in individuals with existing heart disease and underlying rhythm disturbances.

  - Alters coagulation factors and makes blood more likely to clot and produce a heart attack.

  - Elevates heart rate, causes arteries to constrict and increases the risk for blockage of coronary blood flow.

  - Increases the risk for high blood pressure and decreases the ability to control high blood pressure once it has occurred. This increases the chances for the development of further cardiovascular disease, stroke and kidney failure.

  - Reduces the levels of the neurotransmitter serotonin, increasing the risk for depression and/or anger as well as the risk for cardio-vascular disease.

  - Signals the body to release fat into the blood, raising blood cholesterol levels and making a heart attack or stroke more likely.

- **Diabetes mellitus, Type II**

  The first signs of the presence of type II (maturity onset) diabetes mellitus may become manifest after acute and/or chronic stress. And, once present, continued stress may make diabetes more unstable and difficult to control because of the continued release of stress hormones and/or the failure of the relaxation response.

- **Depression**

  Depression may result from untreated chronic stress, and may also mimic some of the symptoms of stress including changes in appetite, sleep and concentration. However, it is distinguished from stress by feelings of hopelessness, loss of interest in life, and at times, thoughts of suicide.

- **Eating problems**

  Stress can have varying effects on eating, and cause eating disorders and weight gain or loss. Eating disorders, including anorexia nervosa and bulimia, are associated with maladaptation in response to stress and underlying emotional issues.

  ➢ **Weight gain**

    Overweight and obesity frequently are related to stress. Many people use food as a tranquilizer (comforter) and overeat, and thus gain weight. Men and women who gain weight in response to stress tend to be less able to adapt and manage stress. Release of the stress hormone, cortisol, appears to promote the deposition of abdominal fat, a predictor of diabetes and cardiovascular disease.

  ➢ **Weight loss**

    Stress also causes some individuals to suffer a loss of appetite, decreased food intake, and weight loss. And, rarely stress may cause the thyroid gland to become hyperactive, stimulating appetite and the body to burn calories excessively, resulting in weight loss.

➤ **Gastrointestinal disorders**

The human brain and intestine respond to many of the same hormones and nervous system neurotransmitters such as serotonin. Thus, it is not surprising that chronic stress can cause bloating, constipation, cramping, diarrhea and heartburn.

➤ **Inflammatory bowel disease**

Long-term stress is reported to triple the rate of flare-ups of inflammatory bowel disease (Chron's disease and ulcerative colitis). However, stress is not considered to be a cause of inflammatory bowel disease.

Irritable bowel syndrome (spastic colon) is strongly correlated with stress. In this condition, the large intestine becomes irritated and contractions become spastic rather than smooth and wave-like. The abdomen bloats and the patient has intestinal cramping, alternating with periods of constipation and diarrhea. Sleep disturbances, due to stress can further exacerbate irritable bowel syndrome.

➤ **Peptic ulcers**

H. pylori bacteria and the use of nonsteroidal anti-inflammatory (NSAID) medications (such as aspirin and ibuprofen) now are considered to be primary causes of peptic ulcers. However, research still shows that chronic stress may predispose some individuals to peptic ulcers, or at least sustains existing ones in up to 30–60% of cases, mandating attention to psychological factors in the majority of cases.

• **Immune disorders**

Stress can have mixed effects on the immune system and autoimmune disorders. For example:

➤ Short term stress appears to have little or no effect on multiple sclerosis but under chronic stress, the risk for flare-ups increases.

➤ Eczema, lupus, and rheumatoid arthritis may improve or deteriorate in response to stress.

Chronic stress decreases the immune response and increases the risk for infections. Studies indicate that individuals under chronic stress:

➢ are more likely to have a higher incidence of infections;

➢ are more susceptible to herpes or HIV virus activation;

➢ demonstrate impaired response to immunizations;

➢ have low white blood cell counts and are vulnerable to upper respiratory infections and colds;

➢ progress more rapidly to AIDS from HIV status.

- **Memory, concentration and learning**

Stress produces significant effects on the brain, particularly as regards memory, concentration and learning. A more or less immediate effect of acute stress is an impairment of short-term memory, particularly verbal memory. The typical victim of severe acute stress usually suffers not only from memory loss but also from loss of concentration at work and at home, becoming inefficient, accident prone and suffering from inhibition of learning and recall. All this may be due largely to the effect of stress hormone. Fortunately memory loss, concentration and learning ability usually are restored after the relaxation response occurs.

Chronic stress is reported to be linked to shrinkage in the brain's hippocampus area, the center of memory. Studies have shown that groups of Vietnam veterans suffering from post-traumatic stress disorder, and sexually abused women, have displayed shrinkage of the hippocampus. Whether or not such shrinkage and corresponding memory loss is reversible or not remains to be demonstrated.

- **Pain**

Chronic muscular and joint pain caused by arthritis and other conditions may be intensified by stress. Psychological distress also is reported to play a significant role in the severity of neck and back pain. Job dissatisfaction and depression are linked to back pain problems. Tension headaches and migraines commonly are associated with stress.

- **Sexual and Reproductive Dysfunction**
  - ➤ **Sexual function**

    Diminished sexual desire and inability to achieve orgasm occurs frequently in women under stress. Temporary impotence in men may also result from stress. Release of catecholamines, as a result of the stress response, constrict the smooth muscles of the penis and its arteries reducing blood flow into, and increasing blood flow out of, the penis which can prevent a sustained erection.

  - ➤ **Fertility**

    Stress hormones have an impact on the hypothalamus and may affect fertility, shut down or shorten menstruation and increase pregnancy loss, especially in women with stressful jobs.

    Maternal stress during pregnancy has been reported to be associated with:

    - increased incidence of premature birth;
    - increased infant mortality;
    - lower birth weights;
    - risk of miscarriage.

- **Skin Disorders**

  Stress plays a significant role in exacerbating a number of skin conditions such as ezema, hives, psoriasis, and rosacea. Excessive itching of the skin may also be caused/exacerbated by stress.

- **Self Medication and Unhealthy Lifestyles**

  Individuals under chronic stress frequently seek relief through drugs, alcohol, smoking, comfort eating, or more passive activities such as watching television excessively. The damage caused by these unhealthy self-destructive habits is compounded by the physiologic effects of stress itself. And the cycle is self-perpetuating since a sedentary routine, an unhealthy diet, alcohol and/or drug abuse, and smoking promote disease, interfere with sleep, and lead to increased, rather than reduced, stress/tension levels. Drinking five or more cups of coffee, for example, can cause changes in blood pressure and stress hormone levels similar to those produced by chronic stress. An unhealthy lifestyle is one of the chief causes of stress and chronic diseases.

- **Sleep Disturbances**

  Unresolved stress frequently causes insomnia, keeping the stressed individual awake or causing awakening in the middle of the night or early morning.

- **Teeth and Gum Diseases**

  Stress has now been implicated in increasing the risk for periodontal disease, a disorder of the gums that is now recognized as a significant risk factor for cardiovascular disease.

- **Unexplained Hair Loss**

  Alopecia areata is unexplained hair loss in a localized patch of the scalp. The cause remains unknown but stress is believed to play an important role. Hair loss often occurs during periods of intense stress such as mourning.

Additional information on stress is available at:

- Mayo Clinic

  Signs and Symptoms of Stress: Prompt Recognition is Crucial

  http://www.mayoclinic.com/health/stress-symptoms/SR00008_D

  Stress: Why You Have It and How It Hurts Your Health

  http://www.mayoclinic.com/health/stress/SR00001

1.11   Relaxation Response: Resolution of Stress

Once the threat/demands of stress have been met/resolved, the body's systems normalize and the resolution of stress occurs. This is known as the relaxation response.

Chapter 2 — Stress Risk Factors

Individuals respond differently to stress depending upon certain factors that may play an important role in initiating stress. Some of the more important factors include:

2.1   Abusive Behavior

Abusive behavior towards children may result in long-term abnormalities in the HPA system and the relaxation response, which regulate stress. And, while no one is immune to stress, it may simply go unnoticed in the very young until it has taken its toll.

Aggressive or depressed mothers may be significant, influential sources of stress in children, an even more important factor than poverty and over-crowding. Children become frequent victims of stress because they often are unable to express their feelings or communicate effectively regarding their responses to events over which they have no control. Girls tend to become stressed from interpersonal situations, and stress is more likely to lead to depression in girls than in boys. For boys, changing schools or poor grades appear to be the more important sources of stress. And the probability of childhood behavioral difficulties in a boy appears to increase with the number and type of stressors encountered in the home.

2.2   Angry Personalities

Angry personalities who are less emotionally stable or have high anxiety levels tend to experience events as more stressful than other persons. The exaggerated negative response to stress that such individuals express has been characterized as "catastrophising" the event (turning a stressful event into a perceived mental catastrophe). Such an overly angry or hostile response to stressful situations is known to be particularly dangerous to the cardiovascular system in terms of leading to a heart attack or stroke.

2.3   Caregiving

Numerous studies show that caregivers of physically or mentally disabled family members are at significant risk for chronic stress and its consequences for health. Spouses caring for a disabled partner are particularly vulnerable to a range of chronic stress-related health disorders such as anxiety, cardiovascular disease, depression, diabetes, influenza, and even poorer survival rates. Wives experience significantly greater stress from caregiving than husbands and tend to feel more negative about their husbands.

Some risk factors that tend to put caregivers at higher risk for chronic stress and stress-related illnesses include:

- being a health professional
- highly dependent patient
- high job demands
- living alone with patient
- minority group member, e.g., African-American

2.4   City Dwelling

Individuals who live in cities tend to suffer from higher stress levels.

2.5   Chronic Exposure to Stress

The longer the duration and more intense the stressors, the more harmful the health consequences.

2.6   Divorced or Widowed

A number of studies indicate that divorced or widowed individuals suffer more from chronic stress and its consequences.

2.7   Genetic Factors

Some individuals have genetic factors that affect stress such as having a less efficient relaxation response or an abnormality in serotonin regulation that is associated with heightened reactivity of the heart rate and blood pressure response to stress.

2.8   Immune Disorders

Certain diseases such as eczema or rheumatoid arthritis, due to immune system abnormalities, may actually impair the response to stress.

2.9   Isolation

Isolated individuals suffer from higher stress levels and health consequences.

2.10   Mothers Who Work

Working mothers, regardless of whether they are single or married, undergo higher stress levels and adverse health effects due to a greater work load than other women or men. Such stress may also have a harmful effect on her children.

2.11   Racial or Sexual Discrimination

Those who are the targets of any form of perceived real or imagined racial or sexual discrimination face increased levels of chronic stress and health consequences.

2.12   Relaxation Response Failure

In some individuals stress hormones remain elevated chronically instead of returning to normal levels due to a primary relaxation response failure. This may occur in highly competitive sports athletes, individuals with a history of depression and in other stress-related disease states.

2.13   Social Network Deficiency

Lack of an established network of family and friends predisposes one to stress and stress-related disorders. Older parents who maintain active relationship with their adult children minimize the adverse consequences of chronic stress and stress-related health problems, especially in the lower income and social classes. Individuals who live alone are unable to effectively relieve their stress by having someone close to discuss their negative circumstances and feelings.

2.14   Uneducated, Unemployed, Uninsured

These individuals face increased levels of stress in their lives and stress-related health issues.

2.15   Work

Up to 50% of American workers describe their jobs as stressful and job-related stress is particularly likely to become chronic in such cases because it is such a large part of daily life. Stress reduces a worker's effectiveness and productivity by impairing memory, concentration, learning, and sleep—increasing the risk for stress-related accidents and disease.

Work stress is known to lead to harassment or even violence on the job. Stress that places such a burden on the cardiovascular system, may produce high blood pressure, heart attack or stroke, and may be fatal. In fact, a number of studies now indicate that job-related stress is as great a threat to health as overweight and obesity, not exercising and smoking. The Japanese even have a word for death due to overwork—karoushi.

Key stressors at work may include the following:
- excessive time away from home and family
- ineffective conflict resolution between workers and employer
- lack of effective communication
- lack of job security
- little or no participation in decisions affecting one's responsibilities
- long work hours
- office politics and conflict among workers
- overwork
- unreasonable demands for performance
- wages not commensurate with levels of responsibility

2.16   Worries, Real or Imagined

Real or imagined negative worries/self-talk constitute a major source of stress in life.

Chapter 3 — Happiness, Unhappiness and Stress

3.1   Purpose of Life

The question of the purpose of human life has been raised countless times over past centuries. And, the answer still remains illusive as far as any consensus is concerned.

"Once again, only religion can answer the question of the purpose of life. One can hardly be wrong in concluding that the idea of life having a purpose stands and falls with the religious system."

Sigmund Freud
Civilization and its Discontents, 1930

On the other hand, the question of what individuals themselves show by their behavior and beliefs to be the purpose and intention of their lives— what they demand and wish to achieve in it can hardly be in very much doubt. They strive after happiness and want to become happy and remain so whatever that may mean to each of them.

Individuals with a clear and firm purpose in life appear to achieve the greatest degree of success and happiness.

Dr. Robert Schuller in his book, *Don't Throw Away Tomorrow* (Harper, San Francisco, 2005) emphasizes the importance of having a purpose/mission in life in the three quotes below:

"Discover and determine your mission in life. Everyone needs a mission that will give purpose and meaning to life. The human spirit has an inextinguishable hunger for a cause so consuming that it can fill the emptiness of the soul with pride, purpose, and pleasure. My mission statement keeps me focused on the meaning and purpose of my life and helps me stay on course through the evolving challenges and accomplishments of this process calling living."

"Stay focused on your dreams. Faith plus focus follow through equals mission accomplished. Goals reached, desires fulfilled, vision experienced, mission accomplished, dreams coming true: however you put it, the secret in making success happen is often found in this one discipline "focus—focus on focus".

"Choose positive values that empower your future. Your values will shape your destiny."

Albert Schweitzer also provides words of wisdom on the importance of purpose in life.
"I do not know what your destiny will be, but one thing I can be certain—the only ones among you who will be truly happy are those who sought and found how to serve".

3.2   Happiness and Unhappiness

"Happiness", according to William James, a notable 19th century philosopher and psychologist, "may be estimated by the ratio of one's accomplishments to one's aspirations". And, current research suggests that happiness is greatest when one combines frequent numbers of good events/experiences with less frequent unpleasant ones.

Good events/experiences may be said to include such things as:

- achieving financial independence/stability
- being involved in an interesting, meaningful, productive job
- having a loving, caring spouse or partner
- leading a healthy lifestyle and having good health
- pursuing interesting, pleasurable career and hobbies
- rewarding family and other relationships

More intensely pleasant events/experiences may include such things as:

- birth of a child
- enjoying a rich and meaningful spiritual experience(s)
- helping children grow up, mature, and become successful
- special romantic getaways
- special recognition for personal or professional accomplishments
- winning the lottery

In a recent survey from the August 2006 issue (p. 131) of Money Magazine, of "what makes up the good life", people stated that they tend to favor health and home over things as indicated in the table below:

What Makes Up the Good Life

No.	Percent Favored	Aspect of Life Favored
1	84%	good health
2	60%	a home one owns
3	48%	children
4	46%	an interesting job
5	36%	free and leisure time
6	22%	a yard or garden
7	19%	a luxury or second car
8	19%	latest electronic gadget

However, the happiest people:

- don't waste time dwelling on unpleasant things;

- tend to interpret ambiguous events in positive ways;

- aren't bothered by the successes of others;

- spend less and appreciate what one has more;

- count their blessings and are grateful.

Performing gratitude exercises helps focus the mind on what really matters in life.

Research indicates that to "feel happy", one generally should focus on the frequency and not the intensity of positive events/experiences in our lives and minimize the negative ones as much as possible. Also, placing too great an emphasis on the more intense pleasures of life can easily result in disappointments and disillusionment.

To be unhappy for a long period of time, for whatever reason, may result in chronic stress and its health consequences. Seeking and cultivating happiness in a low stress lifestyle on the other hand, may allow one to effectively cope with, and reduce distress.

3.3   Happiness—Research Findings

Studies and expert opinion regarding happiness appear to indicate that:

- "True" happiness is generally regarded as an enduring sense of positive well-being and an ongoing perception that life is fulfilling, meaningful and pleasant.

- The current, generally accepted idea of happiness is not only too materialistic but also too individualistic. It is better to value close relationships, to be sensitive and compassionate, and responsive to others, to give and receive support, and to be interdependent and not just independent.

- The description of what generally makes people happy has remained remarkably consistent over the past years. This includes health, productive and interesting work, decent income, and loving family and friends, resulting in satisfaction and peace of mind.

- Happiness generally is perceived as a function of the perceived gap between what one has and what one thinks he or she should have in terms of what others have.

- Engaging in work that takes advantage of an individual's strengths and skills, and allows one to strive towards a goal usually makes one feel fulfilled and happy.

- The best predictors of happiness are physical health, income (compared with our family members and friends of a similar age), education, marital status, and spiritual outlook.

- Basic things that may increase happiness and joy in everyday life include:
  - being of service to someone
  - developing a healthy lifestyle
  - expressing gratitude for your blessings each day
  - communicating often with a loved one
  - listening to music you like
  - loving and be loved in return
  - making and enjoying time with friends
  - planting something and nurturing it
  - saying hello to a stranger at least once a day
  - smiling as often as possible

- Individuals generally consider themselves to be the cause of positive events/experiences in their life, control their occurrence, and play a major role in the good things/experiences that happen to them.

- Sense of mastery over both good and bad events/experiences in one's life appears to contribute to an overall sense of well-being/happiness.

- Age and education show only small correlations with well-being/happiness.

- Married people report greater well-being/happiness than single people.

- Trying to ignore negative events/experiences, or simply forgetting about them after they have occurred, does not diminish or remove their unhappy effect.

- Extraversion, or outgoingness, also seems to be strongly associated with happiness. Extroverts are happier even when left alone compared to introverts.

- While physical attractiveness is one of the most highly prized attributes in Western civilization, it only weakly correlates with feelings of well-being and happiness.

- Intelligence shows virtually no correlation with happiness levels.

- An individual's level of happiness may largely be determined by comparisons made with society's standards, social comparisons, on a particular individual's aspiration, past or ideals. If an individual exceeds these standards, he or she may feel happy, otherwise falling short of these standards, a feeling of unhappiness may result.

- The most important factor for feeling happy is good interpersonal relations with a spouse, family members, friends and superiors at work or school, and neighbors.

- Happy individuals often find themselves absorbed in tasks or hobbies they find challenging, and they seek work and leisure that more fully engage their skills.

- Exercise helps relieve anxiety, depression, stress/distress and unhappiness.

- Mutual support and self-disclosure in committed relationships tend to decrease misery and unhappiness.

- If married, it is important to nurture the relationship and not take one's partner for granted. Also, one needs to display the sort of kindness that one wishes displayed to oneself and lovingly share together for a deeper and more enduring happiness.

- Having a faith that provides a support community, a sense of life's meaning, and a reason to focus beyond oneself and life's temporary ups and downs, provide for a more profound level of happiness.

- Surveys indicate that happier individuals generally:

  - ➢ are positive/optimistic and have better self-esteem

  - ➢ become involved in a faith that entails communal support, purpose, self-acceptance, outward focus, and hope

  - ➢ choose challenging, interesting work and leisure

  - ➢ develop feelings of self-control

  - ➢ engage in supportive relationships that allow companionship, confiding and trust

  - ➢ enjoy fitness and have healthier bodies

  - ➢ have more realistic goals and expectations

  - ➢ incorporate music into their lives

- Once basic needs are met, having more money provides diminishing emotional dividends and happiness. An increase in income or possessions beyond the basic needs, may make one feel happy temporarily: however, one soon adapts and begins looking for a "larger fix". Contrary to popular opinion, there is only a modest correlation between income and happiness, and it is much less than most people imagine.

3.4   Love

To love and be loved in return remains one of the keys to true happiness.

Love passed through the prism of St. Paul's inspired intellect and written in the Holy Bible, Corinthian's Chapter 13 may be regarded as having nine aspects. These are patience, kindness, generosity, humility, courtesy, unselfishness, good temper, guilelessness and sincerity.

Patience is a normal attitude of love, waiting to begin, not in a hurry, calm, ready to do its work when the summons comes. Love understands and therefore waits.

Love is "active kindness". The happiness of those about us is affirmed by our being kind to them. Any good thing that can be done, or any kindness that can be shown to any human being, let it be done now. Let it not be deferred or neglected.

Generosity should not include the envying of the generosity of others.

Humility puts a seal upon one's lips to forget what has been done. Love hides from self-satisfaction—being "puffed up".

Courtesy is said to be love in little things such as politeness and behavior which is not unseemly.

Unselfish means not to seek things for oneself because there is no greatness in things—the only greatness is unselfish love. It is more blessed and happier to give than to receive.

Good temper signifies that "love is not easily provoked". A bad temper is not only unloving but is one of the most destructive elements in human nature being made up of jealousy, anger, pride, selfishness, cruelty, self-righteousness, touchiness, and sullenness—all ingredients of a dark and unloving soul.

Guilelessness constitutes a secret of personal influence. "Love thinketh no evil", imputes no motive, sees the bright side of things, puts the best construction on every action. The people who influence you are the people who believe in you. Respect of another is the restoration of self-respect one has lost.

Sincerity stands for "love rejoiceth not in inequity, but rejoiceth in the truth". Sincerity of purpose endeavors to see things as they are, and rejoices to find them better than suspicion feared and refuses to take advantage of another's faults.

Bear in mind that the nine key aspects of love are only that—love itself can never be defined—it remains a mystery in an enigma. It is much more than the sum of its parts/elements.

3.5   Pursuit of Happiness

In the pursuit of happiness, it is considered wise to follow certain principles.

"In a pursuit of happiness, do not quarrel with your lot and station in life. Do not complain of life's never ceasing worries, a petty environment, vexations that you must tolerate, or the small and sordid shoulds that you have to live and work with. Above all, do not resent temptation or be perplexed by life. Through life's practices concerning emotional problems of everyday day living, you need to learn to become patient, humble, generous, unselfish, kind, courteous and sincere—and loving. Do not grudge the hand that is molding the more or less shapeless image within you adding to its ultimate near perfection. Keep in the midst of life as it is—do not isolate yourself—be among people, things, troubles, difficulties and obstacles. Remember: talent develops in solitude, character in the stream of life—the talent of prayer, faith, meditation, of seeing the unseen—whereas character grows in the mainstream of the world's life where one learns to love and be loved in return."

Wolfgang Goethe *Psychology of Happiness*

Old wisdom and recent research indicate that the key to understanding true happiness appears to lie chiefly in our internal qualities and character strengths rather than in external events. In addition, we appear to be able to use these qualities and work with them to help make ourselves "happier" over the longer term.

Studies indicate that true happiness appears to be most strongly associated with a core subset of traits labeled "heart strengths"—gratitude, hope, zest for living, and the ability to love and be loved in return. And loving relationships with other people appear to constitute the basis for making the vast majority of us the happiest.

Most of us focus on our weaknesses and on what we don't have. It is better to reverse the focus from what you did wrong to what you did right, emphasizing strengths to change the way you feel—to much happier. Focusing on gratitude enhances happiness more than any other focusing technique.

3.6   Psychiatrists, Physicians and Antidepressants Do Not Cure Unhappiness

Sigmund Freud once described the goal of psychotherapy as "transforming hysterical misery into ordinary unhappiness". And now, many doctors appear to see it as their mandated duty to eradicate ordinary unhappiness completely with prescription antidepressants and other drugs. However, when drugs are used in the attempt to banish unhappiness, much is lost, especially in children.

A desperate search for happiness appears to have led medicine to enter the realm of the soul, and many doctors are now conflating everyday unhappiness with genuine disease—major depression. And, in so doing, they may have created a new class of so-called "artificially happy people", a societal tragedy.

The catchall word depression unfortunately has lost much of its meaning since it now appears unwisely to cover a wide range of feelings such as ordinary sadness, dejection, disappointment, dissatisfaction and even unhappiness. And, all such unpleasantness is now even regarded as a "condition" in the minds of many doctors that calls for antidepressant treatment.

The opposite of depression is not happiness. In "artificial happiness", people on antidepressants may become complacent about their miserable marriages and careers, unfulfilling jobs and lives, and hollow existences. As a result, many now on antidepressants have become "artificially happy" and largely without purpose or direction in life.

More than 15% of Americans now use antidepressants and only a small percentage may be truly regarded as significantly clinically depressed enough to warrant antidepressant therapy. And, unfortunately, neither psychiatry nor antidepressants can cure unhappiness or produce "true" happiness.

For further information, the reader is referred to the recent book entitled, "Artificial Happiness" by Ronald W. Dworkin, 2006.

3.7   Gratitude, Stress Reduction, and Happiness

Gratitude is an affirmation of the goodness in one's life and the recognition that the sources of this goodness lie chiefly outside the self. The expression of gratitude in one's life is one of the best ways to overcome the failings of a "bad attitude", one of the most stressful and destructive forces in life.

There is no quick fix on the road to gratitude. One way is to seek the Grace of God. It has been said that: Attitude plus the Grace of God results in Gratitude. Another way to become grateful is to act like a grateful person over and over again. With practice, one may eventually become a truly grateful person.

The wisdom of gratitude and "fixing wrong attitudes" may be found in the sayings of the sages of all the ages. Selected from the many, many available, below are a dozen pertinent ones to illustrate this wisdom along with those to whom they are attributed.

Gratitude's Wisdom

1. The greatest discovery of my generation is that a human being can alter his life by altering his attitudes. William James

2. Could we change our attitude, we should not only see life differently but life itself would become different. Katherine Mansfield

3. To be wronged is nothing unless you continue to remember it. Confusius

4. Let us rise up and be thankful, for if we didn't learn a lot today, at least we learned a little, and if we didn't learn a little, at least we didn't get sick, and if we got sick, at least we didn't die; so let us all be thankful. Buddha

5. He who has so little knowledge of human nature as to seek happiness by changing anything but his own disposition will waste his life in fruitless efforts. Samuel Johnson

6. Attitude is a little thing that makes a big difference. Winston Churchill

7. I had the blues because I had no shoes until upon the street, I met a man who had no feet. Ancient Persian Saying

8. Things work out for the better for the people who make the best out of the way things turn out. Art Linkletter

9. Become a possibilitarian. No matter how dark things seem to be or actually are, raise your sights and see possibilities—always see them for they are always there. Norman Vincent Peale

10. A drop of honey catches more flies than a gallon of gall. Abraham Lincoln

11. We plant seeds that will flower in our lives, so best remove the weeds of anger, avarice, envy and doubt. Dorothy Day

12. When you feel "dog tired" at night, it may be because you've growled all day long. Anonymous

3.8   Five Roads to Happiness

When psychologists speak about happiness, they are usually referring to a sense of deep contentment. And, there appear to be five principal roads to achieving deep contentment and the majority of satisfied people pursue all five.

- The first is to have a life full of good times, pleasure and an interesting job.

- The second is to have an engaged life in which you lose yourself to some passion or activity, experiencing "flow".

- The third is to pursue a meaningful life, filled with purpose, but not necessarily with many high moments or blissful experiences, and love and be loved in return.

- The fourth is to pursue a life of sincere gratitude for all your blessings. All happy people are grateful. Ungrateful people cannot be happy.

- The fifth is to be of service and help make the world a better place.

And, it is important to remember that a person can have a great life, be happy, and not necessarily be smiley-faced all the time. Using your character strengths helps compensate for weaknesses or vulnerabilities that otherwise can interfere with happiness.

Relationships with other people are what appear to make us the happiest—constituting the foundation of humanity. And relationships are built on the ability to love and be loved in return. But love doesn't necessarily mean romance. Relationships with other people include friends, parents, children, neighbors, colleagues, co-workers, and others. When we are engaged with fellow human beings and pets we are the happiest.

"Too often we underestimate the power of a smile, a kind word, a listening ear, an honest compliment, or the smallest act of caring, all of which have the potential to turn a life around." Dr. Leo Buscaglia

The word "happy" is derived from an old Norse word, happ, meaning chance or luck; the word "hapless", from the same root, means unfortunate. Until the past two centuries, happiness was considered a gift of God, people could pursue it, but they couldn't will it. In more recent times it is considered to be "mind over matter" as pointed out over 50 years ago in Norman Vincent Peale's best-selling book, "The Power of Positive Thinking" in which he declared "You can think your way to success and happiness".

Happiness

We get happiness by giving it.
If there is a secret to happiness
It is not in doing what one likes to do
But in liking what one has to do.
Happiness is not a thing, but a relation,
A relation between our condition
And what we think our condition ought to be.

Thankfulness is an attitude,
Another name for happiness.
To be thankful means
That one thinks he is better off
Than he deserves to be.

Thus, the road to happiness lies
In changing our thoughts
Not our things.
The human heart is a great green tree,
And when we hang there gifts for others,

We hang up also
Gifts of happiness for ourselves.
For those who bring sunshine
Into the lives of others
Cannot keep it from themselves.

The laws of love, service, of giving
Cannot be evaded or repealed
And who would do either?
It is what we do for others
That we think of most pleasantly.
It is one of God's ways
That all the happiness
That we have brought to others,
Be returned to ourselves
Increased a hundredfold.

Anonymous

The Man in the Glass

When you get what you want in your struggle for self
And the world makes you king for a day,
Just go to a mirror and look at yourself
And see what that man has to say.
For it isn't your father or mother or wife
Whose judgment upon you must pass,
The fellow whose verdict counts most in your life
Is the one staring back from the glass.
Some people may think you a straight-shootin' chum
And call you a wonderful guy,
But the man in the glass says you're only a bum
If you can't look him straight in the eye.
He's the fellow to please, never mind all the rest
For he's with you clear to the end,

And, you've passed your most dangerous, difficult test
If the man in the glass is your friend.
You may fool the whole world down the pathway of life
And get pats on your back as you pass,
But your final reward will be heartaches and tears
If you've cheated the man in the glass.

Anonymous

Self Esteem

Self-esteem is how one feels about oneself as a person—how one judges oneself overall. If one has high self-esteem, one has the appreciation of the full extent of one's personality, accepting oneself for who one is—including both the good and the bad. Good feelings of self-respect, self-love, and self-worth are essential for self-esteem. Feelings of self-worth form the core of personality and the basis of our psychological well-being and remain one of the key determinants of stress levels in life—high self-esteem, low stress levels and low self-esteem, high stress levels, generally.

According to Daniel Goleman in his ground breaking book, *Emotional Intelligence: Why It Can Matter More Than IQ*, says, "Self Awareness—recognizing a feeling as it happens—is the keystone of emotional intelligence—the ability to monitor feelings from moment to moment is crucial to psychological insight and understanding—People with greater certainty about their feelings are better pilots of their lives, having a surer sense of how they really feel about personal decisions."

In this regard, it is important to remember these words of Ralph Waldo Emerson: "What lies behind us and what lies before us are tiny matters compared to what lies within us."

Thus, it is important for one to continuously work on and improve one's self-esteem, self-worth, and be happy now. With good self-esteem, self-worth and the happiness it brings, one can have a good self image.

The reader can find additional information on this subject and how to build one's self-esteem, self-worth in a recently published book entitled "*Healing Your Emotional Self*" by Beverly Engel, 2006.

Character

In our impulsive and compulsive quest for happiness in modern day society, we now have become a throwaway culture. We throw away all sorts of things—appliances, clothes, food and technological gadgets, (last year's cell phone, computer, or electronic device) already are, or are rapidly reaching obsolescence. Technology has become a virtual throw away industry. Trash containers are overflowing and community landfills are becoming mountains as throwaways are added daily. Throwaways also include such things as classical music, time-tested traditions, sexual morality, and religious values—accepting what is for today considered to be fashionable.

Value systems now are confused and conflicted—driven more by primitive, uncivilized passions rather than true and tried values.

Control, ego, money, pleasure, and power are all primeval passions within the human personality. They are an expression of natural emotional drives/hungers in the human psyche shaping our behavior for better or for worse.

True values must transcend these primitive desires and drives as they can compete or divert human resources such as time and energy, from values that build character and ultimately fulfill life with a satisfying self-respect and self-esteem.

Human desires often conflict with values which must define and design our morality. In so doing, values must determine how passions and desires are to be disciplined to promote character development.

As passions are innate emotions, they are distinguished from reason. Values are chosen and form the moral, ethical and spiritual principles that control, direct, guide, manage, and release or restrain our passionate energy. They create enthusiasm and joy, generating energy for life.

When one's personality becomes dominated by negative values, moods may become melancholy, morbid, morose or even mean-minded.

Primitive passions left unmanaged by honorable values permit the individual to become more or less virtually uncivilized. Culture of "anything goes" in marriage, money pursuits, pleasure, relationships or sex, results in "freedom" which verges on cultural anarchy and gives rise to a stressful life. In contrast, a life which thrives on building character allows the individual to lead a much less stressful existence.

Every individual, intuitively, accidentally evolves into a character—a definition of one's personhood—the essential core that defines and describes one's reputation—conceived and born in the arena where one's life's principles are chosen—shaping one's choices and decision in life—the force in one's personality that motivates one to set goals and manage life to meet them. Strong character survives almost any outcome.

"Character is that which can do without success."—Ralph Waldo Emerson

In other words, what one is, is more important than what one does. Great values produce great character. Those devoted to noble and honorable values generally lead less stressful existences.

Religion remains the power of positive spiritual passions. And, no other institution matches the power of religious institutions to mold human personalities with traditional honorable human values.

"Let your conscience write your rules and set your boundaries. Life without a conscience is a river without banks."—Robert H. Schuller

Additional information on happiness is available at:

- American Psychological Association
  Where Happiness Lies
  http://www.apa.org/monitor/jan01/positivepsych.html
- Healthfinder
  The Sweet Smell of Happiness
  http://www.healthfinder.gov/news/newsstory.asp?docid=529756
  With Age Comes Wisdom....and Happiness
  http://www.healthfinder.gov/news/newsstory.asp?docid=533303
- Psych Central
  Life, Liberty and the Pursuit of Happiness
  http://www.psychcentral.com/psypsych/Pursuit_of_happiness
  Happiness
  http://www.psychocentral.com/psypsych/Enjoyment

Chapter 4 — Anger and Stress

4.1   What is Anger

Anger is a normal emotion experienced by everyone. It can range from mild irritation to intense fury and rage. And it can be caused by anything from a friend's annoying behavior to worries about personal problems or memories of a troubling life event. When handled in a positive way, anger can help a person stand up for themselves, fight and overcome injustices. On the other hand, anger can lead to violence and injury when not addressed properly. Law, social norms, and just plain common sense tell us not to lash out physically or verbally every time something irritates us, otherwise, we likely may hurt ourselves and others.

Most normal people experience anger at least a few times a week. Also, it is reported that up to 60% of such anger episodes include yelling or screaming, and less than 10% involve physical aggression which usually is mild and consists of throwing small objects or pushing or shoving someone.

Some individuals with high trait anger have reactions that are more frequent, intense, and enduring, and report more physical aggression, negative verbal responses, drug and alcohol use, and negative consequences to their anger. When anger disrupts or interferes significantly with a sense of self and/or normal daily living routines, this may warrant professional counseling/therapy.

Angry situations usually involve several interrelated dimensions, all operating more or less simultaneously. These include our:

- bodily response to anger;

- experience of anger;

- physiological arousal produced by anger;

- thoughts at the time of anger;

- ways of expressing anger to others.

The bodily response to anger includes:

- stimulus (stressor) triggers the emotion of anger;

- adrenal hormones are released—the stress response;

- breathing rate, heartbeat, and blood pressure rise;

- body and mind give rise to the "fight or flight" response;

- tension/stress builds up.

It is important to remember that anger may not be openly expressed in certain cases but rather remain "masked". Examples of such masked expressions of anger may include:

- Indirect expressions which disguise the anger with sayings as—"I'm not angry" or "I'm just disappointed in you", etc.

- Modified expressions which usually are fairly direct but are expressed in masked form such as: "I'm annoyed", or "I'm fed up", or "I'm ready to explode", or "I was annoyed but not really angry".

- Depression expressions such as "feeling blue" or "down in the dumps". Such expressions are more removed and harder to recognize, and may be indicative of a so-called "masked depressive" episode.

On the other hand, manifest uncontrolled anger, may produce certain serious common problems of everyday living. Two such examples include:

- aggressive driving

- domestic violence

4.2   Aggressive Driving

Aggressive or angry driving has been identified by the public as the number one problem on the roadway today. High profile cases resulting in death and serious injury frequently appear in the news.

NHTSA (National Highway Traffic Safety Administration) defines aggressive driving as the operation of a motor vehicle that endangers, or is likely to endanger people or property due to progression of unlawful driving actions. It may involve:

- excessive lane changing, failing to signal, or failing to see if vehicle movement can be made safely;.
- passing, failing to signal intent, using an emergency lane to pass, or passing on the shoulder;
- speeding or driving too fast for road conditions.

Aggressive Driving is a Traffic Offense

Up to 70% of all traffic accidents annually are caused by aggressive driving such as passing on the right, running red lights and stop signs, and tailgating.

Road Rage is a Criminal Offense

Road rage or angry, excessive aggressive driving is defined as assault with a motor vehicle or other dangerous vehicle.

4.3   Domestic violence

Uncontrollable anger in the form of domestic violence takes a heavy toll on women. Physical abuse such as slapping, hitting, kicking, or forced sex has a stronger impact on health compared with non-physical abuse such as threats, chronic disparaging remarks, or controlling behavior. However, both forms of abuse significantly damage a women's health and often occur together. And, intimate partner violence harms women's physical and mental health even more than do other common conditions such as pain from back disorders and some forms of cancer.

Up to 10–15% of women report some form of domestic violence from their intimate partner. Women recently victimized by domestic violence appear to be up to 4 times more likely to report symptoms of moderately severe depression, and 3 times more likely to be unhealthy in some way.

Interventions that may lower rates of domestic violence include doctors/healthcare providers routinely asking female patients about the issue and when necessary, referring them to appropriate services.

4.4   Intermittent Explosive Disorder (IED)

IED is a little-studied mental illness marked by episodes of angry, potentially violent outbursts like those seen in aggressive driving/road rage or domestic violence (spousal abuse). This disorder may affect up to 7–8% of American adults, 16 to 18 million individuals, in their lifetimes.

People with IED overreact to certain situations with uncontrollable rage, experience a sense of relief during the angry outburst, and feel remorse about their actions afterwards. Over 80% of those with IED may also have concomitant anxiety or alcohol or drug abuse problems, although IED symptoms usually surface first.

Not many individuals with IED are treated for this disorder—most likely because the vast majority of such patients do not believe they have a problem. Instead, they usually believe it is somebody else that has the problem.

Increasing numbers of researchers in the field are now coming to the conclusion that a significant number of cases of aggressive driving, domestic violence and road rage represent IED and should be handled accordingly. It is important to remember that IED individuals have very few coping strategies/abilities and aggression often is a key factor that brings people in for psychiatric/psychological attention. Combination therapy consisting of cognitive-behavior therapy and antidepressants plus mood stabilizers may help IED patients cope with their anger and aggression.

4.5   Self Assessment: Just How Angry Are You?

Self Assessment Chart

The Mayo Clinic provides a self assessment chart for use to determine "just how angry are you?" as well as tips for anger management. This is available at:

- Mayo Clinic

  Anger Management: How Angry Are You

  http://www.mayoclinic.com/health/anger-managemnt/MH00073

If one scores a number of 2, 3 and/or 4 ratings, professional help may be needed to learn how to handle anger in a healthier way. A professional health care provider/physician may be consulted for counseling and/or anger management classes.

Examine Your Anger Patterns

One may also consider professional counseling for anger problems if one:

- angers out excessively and repeatedly;

- experiences reactions such as muscle tension or a racing heart when angry;

- expresses anger in a way that overwhelms oneself or others;

- gets angry enough to hit, throw, or kick things or people;

- gets angry more often than most people;

- hides angry feelings from others or tries to suppress their feelings;

- stays angry for hours;

- uses alcohol or drugs to calm rage;

- uses threatening language or gestures.

One needs to identify the ways anger is expressed in order to determine if changes are needed in dealing with upsetting situations. One may react too aggressively or even too passively. In either case, one can learn new anger management patterns to replace old, unhealthy habits. Anger management is about expressing one's anger in an assertive, acceptable way.

Additional information on anger and anger management is available at:

- Mayo Clinic

  Anger Management: Tips to Control Your Temper

  http://www.mayoclinic.com/health/anger-management/MH00102

4.6 Anger: Effect on Health

When managed inappropriately, anger is likely to negatively affect physical and mental health. Examples of disorders that may develop or become worse if anger is suppressed without an appropriate outlet include:

- aggravation of existing disease/disorder

- cardiovascular disorders

- chronic neck and/or low back pain

- emotional disturbances/mental illness

- endocrine disease/diabetes mellitus
- gastrointestinal disorders
- genitourinary illnesses
- headaches
- nervous system disabilities
- respiratory problems
- skin disorders
- suicidal behavior

A key example of how disease/disorders can interact with anger is given by diabetes mellitus—the perfect breeding ground for anger. It can start with the question "why me". One can go on to dwell on how unfair diabetes is and one may go on to say "I'm so angry at this disease", "I don't want to treat it", "I hate it." Diabetes can make one feel threatened, and when one feels a threat, anger often surges to one's defense.

For more information see:

- American Diabetes Association

  Anger and Diabetes

  http://www.diabetes.org/type-1-diabetes/anger.jsp

Further information on diseases/disorders that may result from, or may be aggravated by, anger is available via searches at:

- Medlineplus

  Search anger related diseases/disorders

  http://www.medlineplus.gov

- Healthfinder

  Search anger related diseases/disorders

  http://www.healthfinder.gov

4.7   Anger Management

Interventions that enable one to manage anger include:

- anger management courses/classes;
- cognitive-behavior therapy;
- communication skills instruction;
- problem solving;
- relaxation/stress management techniques.

Relaxation tools such as deep breathing, progressive muscle relaxation, hypnosis, self-hypnosis, imagery, visualization, tai chi, yoga, and exercise can help one manage anger.

Cognitive-behavioral therapy—changing the way you think and behave in combination with relaxation techniques appears to offer the most benefit in controlling anger. Cognitive behavioral approaches offer ways to help, namely:

- Learn the ABCs of anger

  Helps establish what causes the anger (anger trigger), what can be done about it (behavior), and what happens because of what is done (consequences).

- Identify the triggers causing the anger

  This then allows one to either avoid or confront the provocation.

- Entertain alternate explanations

  Considering alternative explanations of a provoking event allows one to place it in an appropriate perspective and respond properly.

- Clarify expectations

  Anticipate what consequences/events you will encounter.

- Mental rehearsing

  This allows you to create and pattern yourself after positive images you envision.

- Generate more productive thought processes to change behavior

  This makes new actions easier by replacing negative responses to anger with new more positive behavior.

Problem solving enables one to better understand, handle and face the anger problem. Communication, changing one's environment, using humor, and other tips on easing up may prove to be useful as well. Professional counseling may eventually be necessary for the more difficult anger-management problems.

Additional information on anger and anger-management is available at:

- American Psychological Association

  Controlling Anger—Before It Controls You

  http://www.apa.org/topics/controlanger.html

  Advances in Anger Management

  http://www.apa.org/monitor/mar03/advances.html

  Anger on the Road

  http://www.apa.org/monitor/jun05/anger.html

- American Diabetes Association

  Anger and Diabetes

  http://www.diabetes.org/type-1-diabetes/anger.jsp

- Mayo Clinic

  Anger Management: How Angry Are You?

  http://www.mayoclinic.com/health/anger-management/MH0073

  Tips to Control Your Temper

  http://www.mayoclinic.com/health/anger-management/MH00102

- Healthfinder

  Search "anger" and "anger management"

  http://www.healthfinder.gov

- Medlineplus

  Search "anger" and "anger management"

  http://www.medlineplus.gov

Chapter 5 — Caregiving Stress

5.1   Caregiving

Caregivers usually take care of the elderly. Less often caregivers are grand-parents who are raising their grandchildren, or a spouse/partner caring for a loved one who is sick or dying from a chronic disease/disorder. These caregivers usually are not paid to provide the care.

As the American population ages, surveys indicate that the number of caregivers and demands placed upon them will grow. Today, one in four American families, totaling 22 million households, care for someone over the age of 50. And, the number of American households involved in care-giving may reach 40 million by 2007. In addition:

- about 75% of caregivers are women;
- two thirds of caregivers in the US have jobs in addition to caring for another person;
- most caregivers are middle-aged: 35–65 years old.

Caregivers help with many things, such as grocery shopping, house clean-ing, cooking, shopping, paying bills, giving medicine, toileting, bathing, dressing, and eating.

Today, an estimated 45 million Americans serve as unpaid caregivers for the elderly or disabled family members. As healthcare policy veers ever more sharply toward more home and community-based care, the number of caregivers is expected to increase accordingly.

Caring for another person takes a lot of time, effort and work. In addition, most caregivers juggle caregiving with full-time jobs and parenting. In the process, caregivers put their own needs aside, and often report that it is difficult to look after their own health in terms of exercise, nutrition, doctor's visits and medications. So caregivers often end up feeling angry, anxious, depressed, and isolated. And caregiving for people with Alzheimer's disease, cancer, or long term disabilities is particularly stressful and subject to producing caregiver burnout. Studies show that the more hours spent on caregiving, the greater the risk of anxiety, depression, stress, and burnout.

The following may be indicators that caregiving is putting too much stress on one's life:

- change of eating habits—weight gain or loss
- feeling easily irritated, angered or saddened
- feeling tired, fatigued—without energy most of the time
- frequent headaches, upset stomach, other health problems
- loss of interest in hobbies/activities
- sleeping problems—too much or too little

Women caregivers are particularly prone to feeling overwhelmed and subject to caregiver stress and burnout. Studies show that women, in comparison to men, have more caregiving:

- emotional-health problems
- employment-related problems
- stress and burnout

And, individuals who care for their spouses are more prone to caregiving stress than those caring for other family members.

It is important to note that caregiving for another person, when properly handled, also can create positive emotional change. Many caregivers say their role has had many positive effects on their lives giving them a sense of purpose in life. They say that their caregiving role makes then feel useful, capable, and that they are making a difference in the life of a loved one.

5.2   Caregiving Stress

Caregiving stress is the emotional strain and resulting health consequences for the person giving the care. Numerous studies show that caregiving takes a significant toll on physical and emotional health and well-being. Compared with non-caregivers, caregivers are more likely to have health problems and suffer from:

- anxiety and/or depression
- cardiovascular and other diseases
- diabetes mellitus
- significant stress (distress)

Some of the signals that caregivers and their friends and families need to be on the lookout for possible indicators of caregiving stress include:

- anger at the person being cared for
- anxiety/depression
- fatigue/exhaustion
- inability to concentrate
- lack of interest in hobbies/leisure time
- sleep disturbance
- thoughts of harm to self or others
- weight loss or gain

A caregiver who is experiencing any of the above indicators of stress should ask for counseling help from their healthcare provider/physician.

A caregiver can be screened for depression using the free online site located at:

- National Mental Health Association

  http://www.depression-screening.org

Such screening does not make a diagnosis but can help determine whether one should consider seeing their healthcare provider/physician for help.

In addition, if one is a caregiver for a relative or senior citizen, one may contact Eldercare locator at 1-800-677-1116 for information on services that can help manage stress.

Caregivers themselves often have a need for support groups and services because of stress. They can be juggling multiple roles at home and at the workplace. As a result, what now is needed in the healthcare system is reform that would help both the care recipient and the caregiver.

Caregiver Assessment Programs that now are in place in some areas identify family caregivers and their needs so that they can get support and prevent burnout and health consequences.

5.3   Caregiving and Controlling Frustration

Caring for an individual with Alzheimer's disease, or a related dementia, or for anyone with a serious chronic disability for that matter, can be very challenging and overwhelming. Frustration is a normal and valid emotional response to many of the difficulties of being such a caregiver.

While some irritation can be a part of everyday life as a caregiver, feeling significant frustration can have serious health consequences not only for the caregiver but also for the person being cared for. Frustration and distress can negatively impact one's health or cause a caretaker to be physically and/or verbally aggressive toward the loved one being cared for. If caregiving causes significant frustration and/or anger, the caregiver may wish to explore new techniques for coping with a professional counselor.

When frustrated, it is important to distinguish between "what is" and "what is not" within the caregiver's power to change. Frustration often arises out of trying to change an uncontrollable situation/behavior.

Normal daily activities—dressing, bathing, and eating can become sources of deep frustration for the caregiver. Behaviors such as wandering, or asking questions repeatedly can be frustrating and may or may not be controllable behaviors. Unfortunately, the caregiver simply cannot change all frustrating behavior, especially in those suffering from serious disorders such as dementia and other chronic disabilities.

Warning signs of frustration in the caregiver may include such things as:

- anxiety
- depression
- desire to strike out
- increased food or alcohol consumption or smoking
- increased irritability
- lack of patience
- nervousness
- upset stomach

5.4   Prevention and Controlling Caregiving Stress

Dealing with essentially uncontrollable circumstances, the caregiver can control only one thing—how the caregiver responds to the circumstances. The caregiver needs to:

- ask for help when needed;
- calm down physically;
- communicate assertively;
- modify thoughts/attitudes to reduce stress;
- recognize the warning signs of frustration.

One cannot take on all the responsibilities of caregiving by oneself. It is essential that when significant frustration and stress occur, that the caregiver ask for and accept help from others. The caregiver may discuss needs with family members and friends who might be willing to share caregiving responsibilities in an attempt to reduce stress, otherwise a professional may be considered.

5.5   Elder Abuse and Neglect

As the population of older Americans grows, so does the hidden problem of elder abuse, exploitation, and neglect. Every year an estimated 2.1 million older Americans are victims of physical, psychological or other forms of abuse and neglect. And, for every case of elder abuse and neglect that is reported to authorities, experts estimate that there may be as many as five cases that have not been reported.

Elder abuse is a complex problem. Most incidents of elder abuse:

- don't fall into a single pattern;
- happen outside a nursing home;
- involve others beside the infirm or mentally impaired;
- take place at home.

In fact, studies show that elders who are chronically ill, frail, disabled, mentally impaired, or depressed are at greater risk of abuse. And, even those who do not have such obvious risk factors can find themselves in abusive situations and relationships.

Physical abuse can range from slapping, hitting, kicking, shoving, biting to severe beatings and restraining with ropes, chains or devices, causing unnecessary pain or injury. Emotional or psychological abuse can range from name-calling to insulting, intimidating and threatening an individual.

Caregiver neglect can range from strategies that withhold appropriate attention to intentionally failing to meet the physical, social, or emotional needs of the older person. It can include failure to provide food, water, clothing, medications, and assistance with activities of daily living or help with personal hygiene.

Sexual abuse can range from sexual exhibition to rape. It can include inappropriate touching, photographing in suggestive poses, forcing the older person to look at pornography, forcing sexual contact with a third party, or any unwanted sexualized behavior.

Financial exploitation can range from misuse of an elder's funds to embezzlement. It includes fraud, property transfers, purchasing expensive items with older person's money without that person's permission, or denying the older person access to his or her own funds or home.

One of the most difficult problems caregivers face is achieving a balance between respecting an older person's autonomy and intervening before self neglect becomes dangerous. When in doubt, the caregiver should seek appropriate help.

5.6   Relieving Caregiving Stress

Caregivers who work outside the home should consider taking some time off to reduce effects of stress. Taking a break from one's job may help relieve stress symptoms when feeling overwhelmed. Employees covered under the Federal Family and Medical Leave Act may be able to take up to 12 weeks of unpaid leave per year to care for relatives. Consult with your human resources office at work about options for unpaid leave if you are a working caregiver.

Taking care of oneself enables one to become a better caregiver. It is important to make one's health a priority in order to help prevent or relieve caretaker stress by:

- asking and accepting help;

- finding time for exercise and some leisure activities;

- getting enough sleep and rest;

- joining a support group for caregivers in similar situation;

- living one day at a time;

- looking to faith-based groups for support and help;

- staying in touch with friends and family, social activities can help one feel connected;

- using community caregiving resources for support.

5.7   Respite Care

Respite care provides necessary time off for the overworked/stressed caregiver. In the process, respite care reduces caregiver stress and can be provided by:

- adult day-care centers
- assisted living homes
- home health care workers
- short-term nursing home care

This type of care is essential to family caregivers at times. Studies show that respite care helps caregivers keep their loved ones home for longer periods of time and give them better care.

Family physicians now have a systematic approach for assessing the degree of caregiver burden and stress produced. When there are problems, a family physician should be consulted to provide practical counseling about common caregiving stresses and about resources that may benefit caregivers.

5.8   National Family Caregiver Support Program (NFCSP)

NFCSP is a federally funded program through the Older Americans Act. The NFCSP helps states provide services that assist family caregivers. To be eligible for the NFCS, caregivers must:

- care for adults age 60 years, or
- be grandparents or relatives caring for a child under the age of 18.

Each state offers different amounts and types of services. These include:

- caregiving training
- help in accessing support services
- individual counseling and organization support groups
- information about available services
- limited supplemental services to complement the care provided by caregivers
- respite care

5.9   Caregiving Resources in One's Community

Individuals who need help caring for an older person should contact their local area agency on aging (AAA). These are usually listed in the government sections of the telephone directory under "Aging" or "Social Services". A listing of state and area agencies on aging is also available online at:

- Agency on Aging

   http://www.aoa.gov/eldfam/How_To_Find/Agencies/Agencies.asp

The National Eldercare Locator, a toll-free service of the Administration on Aging, is another good resource. They can be reached online at:

   http://www.eldercare.gov

The Eldercare Locator can help find one's local or State AAA.

Many kinds of community care services also are available such as for:

- adult day care
- cleaning and yard work services
- home care
- home modification
- hospice care
- legal and financial counseling
- Meals on Wheels
- senior centers
- support groups
- transportation

There are two kinds of home care: home health care and non-medical home care services. Both types help sick and disabled people live independently in their homes for as long as possible. Caregivers and doctors decide what services are necessary and most helpful.

Home health care includes health-related services such as:

- medicine assistance
- nursing services
- physical therapy

Non-medical home care services include:

- companionship
- cooking
- housekeeping

Medicare and Medicaid and some private insurance companies will cover the cost of limited home care. Coverage varies from state to state. Other times, you will have to pay out-of-pocket for these services. To obtain Medicare home health care, a person must meet all of the following four conditions:

- A doctor must decide that the person needs medical care in the home and makes a plan for home care.

- The person must need at least one of the following: sporadic (not full-time) skilled nursing care, physical therapy, speech language pathology services or occupational therapy.

- The person must be homebound. This means that he or she is normally unable to leave home. When the person leaves home, it must be infrequent, for a short time, to get medical care, or to attend religious services.

- The home health agency caring for the person must be approved by the Medicare program.

To find out if one is eligible for Medicare home health care services, call the regional Home Health Intermediary at 1-800-MEDICARE or visit the Medicare Website at:

   http://www.medicare.gov and search "Helpful Contacts"

In order to qualify for Medicaid, a person must have a low income and few other assets, and Medicaid coverage differs from state to state. In all states, Medicaid pays for basic home health care and medical equipment. In some states, Medicaid will pay for a homemaker, personal care, and other services not covered by Medicare.

For more information on Medicaid coverage of home health care in one's state, call the state medical assistance office. For these state telephone numbers, call 1-800-MEDICARE.

Additional information on caregiver stress is available at:

- Medlineplus

   Search "caregiver's stress"

   http://www.medlineplus.gov

- National Women's Health Information Center

   Caregiver Stress

   http://www.womenshealth.gov/faq/caregiver.htm

- American Family Physician
  A Practical Guide to Caring for Caregivers
  http://www.aafp.org/afp/20001215/2613.html
- Mayo Clinic
  Alzheimer's: Long Term Care Options0
  http://www.mayoclinic.com/health/alzheimers/AZ00028
  Caregiving: Maintain Your Support Network
  http://www.mayoclinic.com/health/alzheimers-cargiver/AZ00018
  Long Term Care for Your Parents: What to Consider
  http://www.mayoclinic.com/health/long-term-care/HQ01517
- American Psychological Association
  Elder Abuse and Neglect: In Search of Solutions
  http://www.apa.org/pi/aging/eldabuse.html

Chapter 6—Family Stress

6.1   Introduction

Family stress, one of the leading causes of stress, can be defined as a real or imagined imbalance between the demands on the family and the family's ability to meet those demands. In other words, if there are stressful events happening to a family over and above that which the family can handle successfully, family stress results.

"By definition, the human soul is attached to life in all its particulars and prefers relatedness to distancing. Our ultimate goal is to find ways to embrace both attachment and resistance to attachment, and the only way to that is reconciliation of opposites.
With all of their inherent difficulties, relationships of all kinds enrich our lives and help fulfill the needs of the soul."

> Thomas Moore, Ph.D.
> *Soul Mates; Honoring the Mysteries of Love and Relationships*, 1993

The demands on the family that are commonly referred to as stressors usually comprising either a life event or a transition that happens to the family. Stressors can be either positive or negative and can cause change in the family's coping pattern. Examples of negative family stressors may include events like:

- children's emotional problems and substance abuse;

- death or serious illness of immediate family member;
- loss of job by breadwinner;
- money/financial problems.

Other stressors such as the birth of a child, job promotion, or graduation of a child can be positive eustressors.

6.2 Aspects of Family Stress

The degree of family stress produced depends upon three major aspects:

- perception;
- resources/family strengths;
- conditions/coping skills.

Perception

How the stressor/stress is perceived has a major determining effect on the resulting family stress. This perception reflects each individual family member's, as well as the entire family's, values including their previous experience in dealing with change and stress. Such may range from seeing the changes as challenges to be met—to the extreme of viewing the stress produced as uncontrollable and the beginning of the destruction of the family.

Resources/Family Strengths

All families have at least some resources and family strengths, some more than others, some within the family and others outside, enhancing the family's ability to cope with stress. These resources/strengths may include such things as:

- common goals and objectives;
- family's ability to solve problems;

- communication skills/patterns;
- financial resources;
- relatives and friends;
- services and support groups in the community.

These may be used to cope with the stress encountered.

Condition/Coping Skills

The family's perception of the stressful event and resources/family strengths all may be useful in coping with stress, minimizing effects, and enhancing ability to prevent a crisis. A crisis usually occurs when behavior patterns are ineffective and new ones are called in, providing families with both dangers and opportunities.

Recognizing Symptoms of Family Stress

One of the best ways to know if a family is experiencing too much stress is through impressions and feelings of family members. They may report the following when questioned:

- bickering/complaining too much;
- communicating poorly and infrequently;
- conversations centered on time and tasks rather than individuals and feelings;
- desire for simpler life;
- escaping into work or other activities;
- explosive arguments;
- little time spent together;
- meals eaten separately or in haste;
- sense of guilt;
- sense of urgency or frustration.

Less-stressed families, on the other hand, tend to:

- communicate regularly and support each other;
- display more flexibility;
- do things and have fun together;
- have more reasonable expectations;
- believe that it is never too late to learn new coping strategies;
- view stress as a challenge that is temporary and controllable.

Also, less-stressed families generally feel that the strategies listed below can help create a less stressful household and allow more time for rewarding interactions among family members:

- avoid being a "superparent";
- give credit for tasks accomplished;
- learn to say no to less important things;
- make lists of things to do together;
- moderate the compulsion to "get it all done yesterday";
- review standards—strive for "excellence" but settle for less when necessary;
- realistic about time frames;
- select commitments judiciously;
- try not to spread family members time too thin.

6.3   Family Changes and Stress

Stress may be regarded as synonymous with significant family change. When the family situation/dynamic changes significantly stress is a consequence. Family change/stressors may include such things as:

- aging parent becomes critically ill;
- breadwinner spouse retires or loses an important job;

- cherished member of the family or friend dies;
- child starts skipping school and "acts out";
- couple enter the "empty nest" syndrome;
- family moves to a new location/city;
- wife goes back to work "to make financial ends meet".

Some families adapt well to such changes and there is little or no significant stress to deal with while others do not and suffer stress accordingly.

Many hold that the home should be a haven of peace and tranquility and that it is acceptable to experience work related, but not family related, stress. The truth is that most families do not measure up to this view since a significant amount of family stress is inevitable in most families. How a family handles and copes with this stress constitutes what is important. And families can develop necessary, effective coping skills for handling such stress.

6.4   Ways to Reduce Family Stress

Research indicates that families managing to reduce and cope with stress in certain ways can be successful. Families that appear to cope most successfully are ones in which members:

- accept and endure hardships;
- accept each others feelings, concerns and ideas;
- develop social support within the community;
- develop their own self-esteem;
- do things as a family;
- don't let problems between each other go unresolved;
- find time to get together often;
- help each other in time of need;
- learn problem-solving skills;

- learn to talk, listen, and communicate with each other;

- let other members know they are understood and loved;

- reach out to friends, neighbors, and community;

- reduce tension and conflict in the family;

- remain close to each other;

- use a range of tension-reducing measures such as exercise, relaxation strategies, positive thinking/optimism, and involvement in family activities (e.g., picnics, vacations, etc.), hobbies, community social events and charities;

- work hard at keeping the family functioning.

It is important to remember that all events which change the family situation, especially the unexpected or undesirable ones, create stress, some more than others. And, family members usually do not anticipate or prepare well for the adaptations all family members have to make when one or more of these stressful events occur.

The number of stressors a family experiences within a given period of time also is important in determining the degree of stress that must be endured. Multiple stressful events occurring at the same time or in a given short period of time, can lead to "stress pile up", greatly increasing the amount of stress to more unbearable levels, and reducing the ability of the family members to cope.

Women are reported to be the chief health-care managers of their families—since 73% of women identify themselves as such according to a recent survey. Thus they bear the brunt of the family healthcare burden of stress. From taking care of their own health to serving as the caregivers for their children, parents, and spouse, each aspect of care brings more stress. And, unfortunately, too often women do not take the necessary steps to cope satisfactorily, and their own physical and mental health suffers accordingly.

Moreover, men and women are reported to exhibit and handle their stress differently—women being more likely than men to report feelings of nervousness, lack of energy, and wanting to cry. Men, on the other hand, who consider themselves the primary healthcare decision makers, are more prone to describing their stress in terms of being angry, irritable, and having difficulty sleeping.

In addition, there appear to be significant gender differences in coping mechanisms used to deal with stress within the family with the effect that:

- over fifty percent of women admit to being "comfort eaters" as a means of handling stress whereas only around twenty percent of men report eating to deal with their problem/stress.

- "comfort eaters", in turn, appear to be more likely to exhibit higher levels of the more common stress symptoms/signs, namely fatigue, lack of energy, nervousness and sleeplessness.

- twenty-one percent of those who eat at a fast-food restaurant report being very concerned about stress compared to a little over ten percent who did not. Not surprisingly, fast food eaters report more serious health problems like cardiovascular disease.

Survey results indicate that stress results from a conglomeration of concerns/stressors, and the key is learning how to cope effectively and manage stress.

Individuals/families who turn to food for comfort, alcohol, smoking, or illegal or prescription drugs, to reduce stress can suffer serious health problems that result in even more stress. Counseling with a psychologist or one's healthcare provider/physician should be considered to help modify such unhealthy habits and lifestyle.

Families can be torn apart by illness, divorce, or other problems that create conflict and stress. Family therapy can help them identify and resolve problems. One's family can be the greatest source of support, comfort and love. However, it also can be one's greatest source of pain, grief, and stress.

A health-crisis, work problems or teenage rebellion may threaten one's family peace and tranquility. Family therapy may help the family cope with such issues as:

- abuse or violence
- conflict
- divorce
- eating disorders such as anorexia or bulimia
- financial stress

- grief, loss and trauma
- illness/health crisis
- marital problems
- parenting skills
- teenage rebellion
- work stress

Family therapy also may be an addition to other types of treatment, particularly for certain mental disorders that require more in-depth treatment.

Additional information on family stress is available at:

- American Psychological Association

  Stressed Out Nation

  http://www.apa.org/monitor/apr06/nation.html

  Americans Engage in Unhealthy Behaviors to Manage Stress

  http://www.apa.org/releases/stresssurvey0206.html

  Lower Family Stress Tied to Improved Child Behavior

  http://www.apa.org/monitor/sep04/lower.html

- Mayo Clinic

  Family Therapy: Healing Family Conflicts

  http://www.mayoclinic.com/health/famly-therapy/HQ00662

- Medlineplus

  Search "family stress"

  http://www.medlineplus.gov

- Healthfinder
  Search "family stress"
  http://www.healthfinder.gov

Chapter 7 — Financial Stress

7.1   Introduction

Surveys have shown that over 50% of all American workers have money problems leading to significant financial stress and health-related issues. With new federal regulation now making it more difficult to file bankruptcy and "wipe away" debt, workers increasingly are feeling the crunch of financial stress.

Stress-induced anxiety over money problems can affect health in a variety of ways including such things as:

- adverse coping—by gambling and/or drinking alcohol excessively, overeating, smoking or using illegal drugs, etc.

- cutting corners in self-care—reducing necessary personal health care and leisure time activities, etc., to help pay for basic necessities like food, rent, etc.

- trouble sleeping—producing a significant sleep deficit that can impair immune function and cognitive abilities.

- unhealthy emotions—as debt piles up, individuals can experience increased anger, anxiety, frustration, and hopelessness which compounds the stress from adverse coping and self-neglect.

Therefore it is no wonder that "money problems" are one of the leading causes of stress in Americans.

Additional information is available at

- About, Inc./New York Times Company

    Financial Stress: How It Effects Your Health and How to Avoid It

    http://stress.about.com/od/financialstress/a/financialstress.htm?

    Addictions and Other Unhealthy Responses to Stress

    http://stress.about.com/od/unhealthybehaviors

Workers financial stress is compounded by the fact that:

- they often fail to properly save for the "rainy days of unemployment" or retirement.

- over 50% worry excessively on how much they owe and are dissatisfied with their financial situation.

- up to one third report that money worries hamper their job performance and family relationships significantly.

- up to 25% of workers in the United States feel they are experiencing stress from financial problems to the extent that productivity on the job is negatively impacted.

Today, surveys indicate that financial stress remains one of the most glossed over worker issues. And, there appears to be substantial costs to the employer caused by lost productivity and stress-related health care costs.

It is estimated that providing personal financial education to workers could save American industry billions of dollars. And the return on investment for the employer for employee financial education can be as high as a ten to one dollar ratio—ten dollars saved for every one dollar invested/spent. Additionally, over 75% of workers report that they have made better financial decisions as a result of personal financial education, and over 50% after workplace financial education.

7.2   Warning Signs of Too Much Debt

Credit is wonderful when it is used judiciously. However, more and more Americans are over their heads in debt which threatens their financial future. Increasing numbers of individuals are running out of credit or becoming enslaved to their debt to the point that it may take up to decades to pay off purchases whose prices have become grossly inflated by high interest charges that accumulate for years. Unfortunately, one's credit card debt is not under control just because one manages to pay monthly minimums and one is not late on any payments. Don't be lulled into a false sense of security by just making minimum credit card payments monthly as continuing this process for a significant period of time may easily lead to a financial crisis.

Some warning signs of serious, stress-producing debt problems include:

- gambling excessively—to attempt to pay off debt
- bouncing checks
- collectors calling for payments
- credit card overused
  - ➢ advances taken to pay other bills
  - ➢ balances at or near limit
  - ➢ payments made are minimum only
  - ➢ purchases declined by credit card company
  - ➢ statements hidden from family, partner or spouse
- increasing amounts of total income needed to pay off debts
- lies to family, partner or spouse about spending excesses
- reverse mortgage taken on home to pay off debt
- savings amounting to little or none

One must first realize that too much debt may produce a significant financial crisis/stress before it is possible to turn finances around and fix the problem. Unfortunately, there is no easy way to do this. However, if one is motivated to get started, a budget, can be used to evaluate income and expenses and can be helpful.

7.3   Budgeting Improves One's Financial Life

The reasons why one should budget include the following. A budget may:

- allow one to sleep better and worry less about how to make ends meet.
- enable one to spend money on things that matter, avoiding unnecessary purchases.
- help you meet your saving's goals.
- reveal areas where you are spending too much money so you can refocus and accomplish more important goals.
- serve as a communication tool in helping bring family members closer together and reducing arguments about money.
- will tell you if you are living "within your means".

7.4   Budget Breakers that May Ruin Your Financial Life

Two key budget breakers that can ruin one's financial life include holiday overspending and compulsive gambling.

Holiday Overspending

Like relationships, one's financial situation can cause stress at any time of the year. However, overspending during the holidays, or anytime for that matter, on gifts, travel, entertainment, along with other non-essentials, can increase financial stress as you try to make ends meet while ensuring that everyone on your shopping list is happy. Thus, financial stress and accompanying anxiety/depression can ruin your holidays and affect your health. Seeking support, instituting proper budgeting and controls, being realistic, and planning ahead can help to ward off holiday financial stress and depression.

Additional information on holiday overspending is available at:

- Mayo Clinic

  Stress, Depression and the Holidays: 12 Tips for Coping

  http://www.mayoclinic.com/health/stress/MH00030

Compulsive Gambling

While approximately 85% of Americans report having gambled at some point in their life, most individuals who gamble are not compulsive gamblers. However, an estimated 2 million plus American adults become compulsive gamblers at some point in their lifetime—losing control of their betting with serious financial consequences first in budget breaking and subsequently in financial stress and the quality of their lives and health.

Additional information on compulsive gambling is available at:

- Mayo Clinic

  Compulsive Gambling

  http://ww.mayoclinic.com/health/complusivegambling/DS00443

Adopting more healthy habits will take you down the road of low stress living. Such ways/habits take a little practice to develop but will be well worth it in the long run in terms of less stress, better health, improved relationships and life satisfaction.

Additional information on a low-stress lifestyle is available in Chapter 9.2.2 and at:

- About, Inc./a New York Times Company

  Tools and Tips for Living a Low-Stress, Healthy Lifestyle

  http://stress.about.com/od/lowstresslifestyle

7.5   Lay the Foundation for Financial Freedom

People with goals succeed chiefly because they know where they are going and how to get there. Failures, on the other hand, believe that their lives are shaped by circumstances and by things that happen to them—by exterior forces beyond their control. Nothing could be further from the truth, especially as pertains to financial stress.

> *"People are always blaming their circumstances for what they are. I don't believe in circumstances. The people who get on in this world are the people who get up and look for the circumstances they want, and if they can't find them, make them."*
>
> George Bernard Shaw

Wise men throughout history appear to agree that the key to financial success is positive thinking and goals.

> *We become what we think about.*
>
> Earl Nightingale

> *If you think in negative terms, you will get negative results.*
>
> Norman Vincent Peale

It has been estimated that if you take 100 individuals in American today who start out relatively even at age 25 who believe they are going to be successful—having a certain eagerness toward life, a sparkle in their eye and an erectness to their carriage, and life seems like a pretty interesting adventure to them—by the time they are 65,

- only one will be truly financially successful;
- four will be financially independent;
- five will still be working, chiefly because they need to;
- thirty-six will be somewhere in between working and independence;

- fifty-four will be broke—depending on others for life's necessities.

"Financial success and failure in life lies chiefly in goals. The difference in outcomes is goals. The person who has little or no goal, who doesn't know where he is going, and whose thoughts must therefore be thoughts of confusion, anxiety, fear and worry will thereby create a life of frustration, fear, anxiety, and worry. And, if he thinks about nothing—he becomes nothing."

Earl Nightengale

Avoiding financial stress necessitates that one must lay the foundations for financial freedom as early as possible in life. One should:

- be clear about potential for any inheritance;
- not count too much on the government or employer pension plans;
- not forget health insurance needs;
- establish a savings plan;
- pay down the mortgage and credit card debt;
- engage in financial planning and budgeting;
- spend less, save more, and invest wisely for growth and income.

7.6   Help is Available Now for Financial Stress

A personal private financial planner can provide you with a plan and the necessary help for handling financial problems.

Your physician, healthcare provider, or psychologist can provide the necessary counseling/treatment for any financial stress and related health problems.

Non-profit agencies/groups are available for credit/debt counseling and other financial problems, such as:

- National Credit Counseling Service
  http://www.familycredit.org
- Money Management International
  http://www.moneymanagement.org
- Gamblers Anonymous
  http://www.gamblersanonymous.com

These agencies/groups can provide services such as:

- budget financial counseling;
- debt reduction/repayment plans;
- credit restoration;
- reduced interest charges;
- stop collection calls and foreclosure on home property;
- financial educational workshops.

Additional information on financial stress is available at:

- About.com/a NY Times Company
  Financial Stress: Managing Your Money—And Your Stress
  http://stress.about.com/od/financialstress
  Financial Tools for Stress Reduction
  http://stress.about.com/od/financialtools
  Stress and the Effects of Money
  http://stress.about.com/library/lifestylequiz/blmoney.htm
  What Stresses You the Most
  http://stress.about.com/library/polls/blstresspoll1.htm
  Financial Stress: How It Affects You and What You Can Do
  http://stress.about.com/od/financialstress/a/financialstress.htm

Chapter 8 — Job Stress

8.1 Introduction

The concept of job stress may be confused with challenge; however, these two concepts are not the same. Challenge energizes us psychologically and physically, and it motivates us to learn new skills and master our jobs. When a challenge is met we feel relaxed and satisfied. Thus, challenge is an important ingredient for healthy and productive work. The importance of challenge in our work lives is probably what people are referring to when they say "a little bit of stress is good for you"—that a little stress/anxiety (eustress) may be regarded as the "creative force of Western civilization".

Job stress, on the other hand, can be defined as the harmful physical and emotional effects that occur when the requirements of the job do not match the capabilities, resources or needs of the worker—leading to decreased productivity, stress-related health problems or injury.

8.2 Economic Impact

Surveys show that around fifty percent (50%) of workers in America are reported to be suffering from significant job stress. In addition, up to 25% of workers report a significant degree of job burnout—a state of physical, emotional and mental exhaustion caused by long-term exposure to demanding work situations. And, stress is considered to be the chief reason for around 70–90% of worker's hospital visits, driving up health care costs. In fact, it is estimated that stress-related illness currently cost companies in America in excess of $200–$500 billion dollars each year due to increased absenteeism, tardiness, decreased productivity, stress-related illness, loss of talented workers, and other factors.

8.3   Causes of Job Stress

Nearly everyone agrees that job stress commonly results from the interaction of the worker and the conditions of work. However, views differ on the importance of worker characteristics versus working conditions as the primary cause of job stress. These differing viewpoints are important because they suggest ways to prevent stress at work.

According to one school of thought, differences in individual characteristics such as personality and coping are most important in predicting whether certain job conditions will result in stress—in other words, what is stressful for one person may not be a problem for someone else. This viewpoint leads to prevention strategies that focus on workers and ways to help them cope with demanding job conditions.

Although the importance of individual differences cannot be ignored, accumulating evidence suggests that certain working conditions in themselves also are stressful to a significant number of workers. In fact, excessive workload demands and working conditions appear to be the source of job stress in many instances, and job design/redesign becomes a primary prevention strategy in those instances.

Workers often cite factors listed below as some of the key causes of stress on the job, namely:
- difficult co-workers;
- inadequate compensation;
- last minute projects to be done a.s.a.p.;

- lean and mean company management;

- limited promotion/career growth;

- overbearing/interfering/micromanaging boss;

- tight deadlines/schedules;

- unrealistic workload.

High pressure work environments take a significant toll on worker morale, well-being, physical and mental health, and productivity.

8.4   Job Stress and Health

Short-lived or infrequent episodes of job stress pose little risk to health. However, when stressful situations go unresolved and become chronic, the body is kept in a more or less constant state of activation by the stress response increasing the rate of wear and tear to biological and mental health systems. Ultimately, fatigue or damage results and the ability of the body to repair and defend itself can become seriously compromised. As a result, the risk of injury or stress-related disease escalates.

Many studies have looked at the relationship between job stress and a variety of illnesses. Mood and sleep disturbances, "upset stomach", headache, and disturbed relationships with family and friends commonly result from job stress. These early signs are usually easy to recognize. However, the effects of job stress in terms of chronic disease take a longer time to develop and can be influenced by many factors other than stress. Nevertheless, evidence has accumulated to show that stress plays an important role in a number of chronic health problems—especially mental, cardiovascular, gastrointestinal, immune system, musculoskeletal, psychological, skin disorders, and sleep disturbances.

8.5   Prevention of Job Stress

Some strategies to help prevent or minimize job stress are as follows:

- attend to the more important and difficult tasks first;
- avoid distractions/interruptions;
- be grateful for the work/job and what it offers;
- delegate workload and minimize micromanaging;
- display sincere loyalty and minimize resistance to authority;
- do not engage in unhealthy coping with stress, seek counseling instead;
- establish necessary controls to be certain tasks are done on time to standards;
- manage expectations;
- organize and prioritize the workload;
- prevent deadline crunches;
- rein in workaholism/schedule work breaks and downtime.

Find ways to be grateful for the work/job and the benefits it may offer.

Remember This—Be Grateful

If you work for a man, in heaven's name, work for him.
If he pays you wages, which supply you bread and butter, work for him;
speak well of him; stand by him; and stand by the institution he represents.
If put to a pinch, an ounce of loyalty is worth a pound of cleverness.
If you must vilify, condemn, and eternally disparage—resign from the
position, and when you are outside, damn to your heart's content but as
long as you are part of the institution, do not condemn it or your boss.
If you do, you are loosening the tendrils that are holding you to the institution, and at the first high wind that comes along, you will be uprooted
and blown away, and probably will never know the reason why.

Anonymous

Stress caused by resistance to authority is one of the key factors that makes working for a boss difficult. This is particularly so for those who feel that they are smarter than their boss. Publicly, and less so privately, diminishing your boss's strengths, overreacting to errors, and resisting and/or resenting authority result in self-inflicted job/career problems. While most problems with authority figures may only represent small day-to-day irritants for the average worker, they can add up to "big time" boss/job dissatisfaction, if one feels and displays that they are smarter than their boss.

On the job, one needs to feel personally valued. Distorting the boss's position in any negative way, makes this much less likely.

Should the boss prevent effective use of your talents, consider leaving the job since some company "out there" is waiting who will better appreciate and use your talents. However, if one realizes that one is standing in one's own way, be smart enough to step aside.

Before deciding to leave your job, do some careful soul searching. First, ask yourself if there is a way to make your current job/career work for you. Can switching to a different department/boss bring new, interesting challenges? Would learning a new skill help one obtain a more interesting position? If the answers are no, then one needs to consider looking for a new job/career.

Remember that although change may go hand in hand with risk, putting up with a job one dislikes can be very stressful—enough to undermine your health. Job stress is associated with an increased incidence of job burnout, headaches, mental disorders, cardiovascular disease, gastrointestinal and immune disorders, skin problems and an unhappy work and personal life.

8.6   Job Burnout

Job burnout is a state of significant physical, emotional, and mental exhaustion caused by a long-term exposure to demanding work situations. If one feels "job burnout", get help, and don't let a demanding job affect your health. According to the Mayo Clinic, one may be prone to job burnout if they:

- find their job to be monotonous;

- identify with work and lack balance between work and their personal life;

- try to be everything to everybody;

- work in helping professions, such as medicine, nursing, counseling, teaching or police work.

If one decides to stay and work things out with the boss and the company, then stress prevention/reduction becomes important to reduce job stress/burnout. The process for a successful job stress prevention program is reported to involve four steps, namely:

- problem identification;

- design and implement intervention;

- evaluate the intervention;

- refine or redirect the intervention strategy as needed.

The best method to explore the scope and source of a suspected job stress problem depends on the size of the organization and available resources. Group discussions among managers, labor representatives, and employees may be all that is needed in a small company. In a larger organization, such discussions can be used to help design surveys for gathering input about stressful job conditions, etc.

Once the sources of stress at work have been identified and the scope of the problem understood the stage is set for design and implementation of an intervention strategy.

Evaluation then is necessary to determine whether the intervention is producing desired effects and whether changes in direction are needed.

The job stress prevention does not end with evaluation. Rather, job stress prevention should be seen as a continuous process that uses evaluation data to refine or redirect the intervention strategy as needed.

8.7   Job Success

Everyone wants some degree of success in life which is largely determined by hard work and choices. A number of people work hard but make bad choices, and it is amazing how many of them believe that they deserve to be more successful because they feel that they have worked so hard.

Working hard is only the first part of success. Making good choices in our working career is the second part, and it truly takes both to achieve success at whatever you do.

Success is not an entitlement—it is not a right or a claim that one should simply obtain—rather success has to be earned through persistent hard work. Failure on the other hand is a choice—failing to meet one's objectives, regardless of what they are, is a choice, because something else has been given higher priority. If one fails—in essence it is because one chooses to fail—and failure is a choice made by the undisciplined and not the self-disciplined.

Discipline involves the act of reaching a goal, and it also reflects the level of commitment that is attached to the goal. Our own various personal commitments are ranked in the order we consciously and unconsciously believe fit with one's life priorities in various stages of life.

Additional information is available at:

- Mayo Clinic

  Work-Life Balance: Ways to Restore Harmony and Reduce Stress

  http://www.mayoclinic.com/health/work-life-balance/WL00056

  Job Burnout: Don't Let a Demanding Job Affect Your Health

  http://www.mayoclinic.com/health/burnout/WL00062

- National Institute for Occupational Safety and Health (NIOSH)

  Work Organization and Stress Related Disorders

  http://www.cdc.gov/niosh/programs/workorgstress.html

- Medlineplus

  Search "job stress" and "job burnout"

  http://www.medlineplus.gov

- Healthfinder

  Search "job stress" and "job burnout"

  http://www.healthfinder.gov

Chapter 9—Stress Management Guidelines and Principles

9.1   Guidelines

An excellent guide for reducing/coping with the stress emanating from the emotional problems of everyday living can be found in the "Serenity Prayer" below:

Serenity Prayer

God Grant me the:
> Serenity to accept the things I cannot change,
> Courage to change the things I can and the
> Wisdom to know the difference.
> Living one day at a time
> Enjoying one moment at a time
> Accepting hardship as the pathway to peace.
> Taking, as He did, this sinful world as it is, not as I would have it.
> Trusting that He will make all things right if I surrender to His will
> That I may be reasonably happy in this life, and supremely happy
> with Him forever in the next
> Amen

Reinhold Niebuhr, 1926

The process of recognizing and coping/adapting to, stress is a life long process, and will not only contribute to better health and a greater ability to succeed, but also to a happier, healthier, and longer life, the ultimate goals sought by many.

Seeking Professional Management/Help

Surveys indicate that up to 60–90 percent of all patient visits are stress-related in at least some measure.

Stress is recognized as an important factor in a variety of physical and emotional illnesses, all of which should be professionally evaluated and treated. A physician should be consulted for any stress symptoms/signs that progress in severity or interfere significantly with every day living.

Certainly consider consulting a mental health professional for any unmanageable stress, especially for severe anxiety, depression, or other mental health disorders. Often, short-term professional counseling can resolve most stress-related emotional problems of every day living.

Considerations in managing stress

Factors that should be considered include:

- combinations of approaches are generally regarded as most effective as no single method is uniformly successful;
- ways that may work for any given individual are not necessarily effective for someone else;
- stress may provide interest, excitement, and motivation for greater achievement while lack of stress may lead to boredom, depression, and demotivation. Thus, stress can be positive as well as negative—and stress reduction needs to be applied accordingly;
- a physician or mental health professional should be consulted if there are any indications of a accompanying stress-related medical or psychological disorder;

- many individuals believe that certain emotional responses to stress such as anger, are innate and unchangeable features of personality. However, research has shown that one can be taught to change unhealthy emotional reactions to stressful events;

- stress management programs cannot cure medical problems and do not substitute for effective medical treatment. However, stress management is of importance in any medical management regime for many diseases. For example, stress management may:

  - reduce psychological distress after a heart attack and improve long-term outlook;

  - reduce the risk of cardiovascular events (e.g. heart attack, stroke) by up to 75% in individuals at risk;

  - be more effective than exercise in reducing cardiovascular disease risks/events;

  - be as effective as antidepressants in treating migraine headaches.

9.2 Principles

Stress management principles include: 1) prevention, 2) adopting a healthy lifestyle and 3) strategies for keeping stress under control.

9.2.1 Prevention

Stress is an essential aspect of life in Western civilization. Prevention or minimization of stress-related disorders is the main goal of stress management.

Most individuals do not pay close enough attention to their health or become aware of the effect of stress/distress in their lives, and the possibility of developing stress-related diseases/disorders. Rather, they tend to deny stress by not recognizing that:

- family history of severe stress/distress is important in determining risk in their own life;

- unhealthy lifestyle is a major factor in the development of stress and stress-related problems;

- the development of significant distress generally is a gradual, lifelong process, and usually cannot be appreciated in the early stages;

- prevention and/or successful coping/adaptation is the best option for success;

- there is a need to take charge, control, and responsibility for one's own stress/distress and do something meaningful about it "before it is too late".

9.2.2 Adopt a Healthy Lifestyle

A key factor in the successful prevention or minimizing of stress lies in the adoption of a healthy lifestyle.

The principles and practices that can contribute to a less stressful and healthier lifestyle are summarized below:

- alcohol use—sparing or not at all

- annual medical check-up—choose a physician and healthcare facility prudently and maintain good health and fitness

- avoid intentional harm to oneself, others or anything

- be grateful for all your blessings: do not take others or things for granted

- communicate effectively with others

- develop/follow your purpose in life

- do good by others and the environment

- do not smoke/avoid secondhand smoke

- eat in healthy, nutritiously sound ways

- engage in monogamous, safe sex within marriage/long term relationship

- exercise regularly, maintain fitness, and engage in good body and mental hygiene daily

- live a moderate life and avoid excesses

- maintain normal weight

- make the world a better place

- minimize procrastination

- practice love, compassion, forgiveness, generosity, gratitude, justice for all, mercy, mindfulness, self-control/discipline, stress management and understanding

- sleep regularly and restfully

Living a healthy lifestyle and preventing or reducing and coping with stress/distress increases in direct proportion to the successful incorporation of the above listed principles and practices into one's life.

A materialistic Western civilization produces its discontents and unhealthy lifestyles. We all have to recognize and adopt a healthier lifestyle in order to adopt/cope with the stress/distress encountered from the emotional problems of every day living, and live a healthier, happier, longer and more successful and productive life.

9.2.3 Strategies for Keeping Stress under Control

There are a number of techniques one can employ to cope with stress overload or avoid it in the first place. Learning how to manage the stress that may come along with any new challenge, good or bad, on a regular basis is helpful. Knowing how to de-stress, and doing it regularly, especially when things are relatively calm, can help one get through the more challenging circumstances that may arrive.

Some of the things that can help keep stress under control include:

- Adding daily pleasant activities and events to your life.

  Make time for recreation and take long weekends away.

- Allowing for and using humor in your daily activities.

  Humor is a very effective way to cope with stress. Laughter not only releases the stress of pent-up feelings but also helps one keep perspective and reduce stress. It is not uncommon for individuals to laugh intensely during tragic events, such as the death of a loved one, and use laughter to help endure the emotional pain.

- Being realistic.

  Don't strive for perfection—only God is perfect. And, expecting others to be perfect can seriously add to your stress levels and put undo pressure on them and you. If you need help, ask for it.

- Build resilience.

  A key to health and happiness is resiliency; coping and standing up to stress—having the mind-set it takes to deal with life's stresses in a peaceful, focused way. Even the busiest skeptics can benefit from simple, mind-calming strategies. Certain individuals adapt quickly to stressful circumstances and take things in stride. They are "cool" under pressure and able to handle problems well as they arise. Researchers have identified certain attitudes and behaviors in individuals that enable them to be resilient even when faced with high levels of stress. Some of these are:

  ➢ believe that you will succeed in life if you keep working toward your goals. Be optimistic.

  ➢ build strong relationships and keep commitments to family and friends.

  ➢ develop a support system that you can rely on and ask for help when needed.

  ➢ don't procrastinate—take appropriate action to solve problems that crop up—practice solving problems and ask for help.

> express gratitude for all your blessings in order to overcome attitudes that bring on stress/distress. Stop complaining.

> participate regularly in activities for relaxation and fun.

> regard change as a challenging and normal aspect of life.

> see setbacks and problems of every day living as temporary and solvable.

> think of challenges as opportunities and stressors as temporary problems, not disasters.

• Develop and use a support network.

Individuals who remain happy and healthy usually have very good social support networks. And, having a pet helps reduce stress and stress-related illnesses.

• Discuss feelings with all concerned.

Anger or frustrations that are not expressed in an acceptable way may lead to lingering hostility, a sense of helplessness and depression. The primary goal is to explain one's needs to a trusted friend in as positive way as possible. Direct communication with another may not even be necessary. Writing in a diary or journal or composing a letter that is never mailed may be sufficient.

Keep in mind that expressing one's feelings solves only half the communication problem. Learning to listen, empathize, and respond with understanding is just as important for maintaining strong relationships necessary for emotional fulfillment and reduced stress.

• Establish realistic goals.

Setting and achieving realistic goals reduces stress. Unrealistic goals increase stress. Keep track of progress.

• Exercise—take care of your body.

Experts agree that regular exercise helps individuals to manage stress. Eat nutritious, healthy foods so that the body obtains the correct nutrients to function optimally. Do not turn to substance abuse or other bad habits to ease stress/distress. Although alcohol or drugs may diminish stress/distress temporarily, relying on such measures to cope with stress actually promotes more stress.

Exercise also is an effective distraction from stressful events. Those who follow an active healthy lifestyle need fewer sick and disability days off compared to sedentary workers. Stress/distress poses significantly less danger to overall health in the physically active and fit individual. A varied and interesting exercise regime is easier to enter and adhere to over the long run. Start slowly as strenuous exercise can be dangerous, particularly in one who is not accustomed to it. Obtain the advice of a physician regarding any exercise program. Also, it is important to recognize that approximately half of all individuals who begin a vigorous exercise program drop out within a year. The key for lasting benefits is to engage in exercise activities that are interesting, challenging, satisfying, and work for you.

- Guided imagery.

  Our bodies react to what we imagine as if it were really happening. Guided imagery uses meditation to magnify this power of suggestion and make it work for us. Listening to guided imagery audiotapes, one can go into a trance-like state and visualize the desired healthy changes wanted in our minds and/or bodies as if they were already happening. If one doesn't have time to visualize a peaceful scenario, a physical cue can be created to use as a shortcut to serenity. If you put your hand over your heart every time you meditate or use guided imagery, eventually just putting your hand over your heart can trigger relaxation. Soon you will have created a "Pavlovian conditioned response" which in the midst of a stressful situation can allow one to be stress-free in seconds.

- Keep perspective—look for the positive.

  Focus on positive thinking and positive outcomes. This helps to reduce tension and achieve goals.

- Learn to relax.

The body/mind's natural antidote to stress/distress is the "relaxation response"—which creates a sense of well-being and calm. One can help trigger the "relaxation response" by learning simple breathing exercises and using them when stressful situations arise. Allow time in your schedule for calming and relaxing activities such as reading a good book, listening to pleasurable music, pursuing a hobby, spending time with a pet, taking a relaxing bath or shower, or meditating.

Combinations of relaxation techniques appear to work best at reducing stress. Relaxing techniques are discussed in more detail in Chapter 10.

- Let a little stress motivate you.

This can help you take action to reach your goal.

- Obtain a good night's sleep.

Obtaining a good night's sleep helps keep your body and mind in "tip top" shape, enabling you to better cope with any negative stressors.

- Positive thinking/be optimistic.

Your outlook, attitude and thoughts influence the way you see things. A healthy dose of optimism, positive thinking and gratitude for all your blessings can help you make the best of stressful circumstances/times.

Be positive, live healthier and longer. The endless stream of thoughts that run through one's mind every day—called self-talk (automatic thinking) can be positive or negative. When such thoughts are mostly negative, one's outlook on life is chiefly pessimistic, and when thoughts are mostly positive, one is likely an optimist. And, studies show that these personality traits—pessimism and optimism—can affect not only stress levels and well-being but also how healthy and long one will live.

In general, having an optimistic, positive outlook in life appears to enable one to better cope with stress while a pessimistic outlook may have an opposite effect. And, optimism reduces stressful negative thinking such as:

- catastrophizing or automatically anticipating the worst;

- filtering—magnifying the negative aspects of any given situation and filtering out the positive ones;

- personalizing—automatically blaming oneself for the negative in life;

- polarizing—seeing things as only either good or bad, black or white—with no middle ground—if one is not perfect, one is a total failure.

One of the biggest differences between optimists and pessimists is their attitudes.

Current attitudes are habits built in ourselves from the feedback of parents, friends, society and self, which form our self-image. These attitudes are maintained by the inner conversation we constantly have with ourselves, both consciously and subconsciously. Thus, the first step in changing our attitudes is to change our inner conversations.

Keep in mind that the things one tells oneself are frequently the real producers of stress, rather than the event itself. So learn to tell yourself the truth and liberate and relish your positive nature, overcoming attitude with gratitude and positive thinking,

Remember, one can learn to turn negative thoughts into positive ones but it takes practice. Thus, try to put a positive spin on as many of your negative thoughts as possible. Optimism enables one to handle everyday stress in a more realistic and constructive way.

Remember, our feelings, beliefs and knowledge are based largely on our internal thoughts. Positive thinking involves dedicated efforts in remembering and repeating the thoughts with positive feelings.

Additional information on positive thinking is available at:

- Mayo Clinic

  Positive Thinking: A Skill for Stress Relief

  http://www.mayoclinic.com/health/positive-thinking/SR00009

- Depression Guide

  Positive Thinking: Power of Positive Phrases

  http://www.depression-guide.com/positive-thinking.htm

- Practice patience.

  Develop the ability to postpone immediate gratification for future gratification—the cardinal sign of emotional maturity and intelligence.

- Reduce/eliminate over scheduling.

  If one is feeling stretched out/overloaded with things to do, consider rescheduling activities, opting to handle only the ones that are considered most important at the time.

- Restructure priorities.

  Shift the balance from stress-producing to stress-reducing activities.

- Solve problems—don't procrastinate.

  Learning to solve the problems of everyday living and managing the stressors of life can give one a better sense of control and responsibility. On the other hand, avoiding or suppressing them can leave one with the feeling of little or no control, making one more anxious, and adding to the stress. Take the time to calmly look at a problem, figure out options, and proceed with action toward a solution. Being capable of solving problems builds inner strengths to handle life's bigger ones—and this can serve one well in times of severe stress/distress.

Chapter 10 — Stress Management — Relaxation Techniques

A number of relaxation techniques are available for stress management. Some considered to be among the more useful are as follows:

10.1 Breathing Exercises

Deep breathing is regarded as a useful stress reliever that "wakes up the brain", relaxes muscles and quiets the mind. It helps to release tension, producing a calming effect and relief of stress. Breathing exercises are regarded as especially useful in stress relief because they are free and you can do them anywhere, de-stressing in a few minutes.

During stress, breathing becomes shallow and rapid. Deep breathing exercises consciously restore breathing to normal, reducing stress. To accomplish this reversal, inhale through the nose slowly and deeply to the count of eight, making sure that the stomach and abdomen expand but the chest does not rise up. Hold the breath for a few seconds and exhale through the nose, slowly and completely, also to the count of eight. To help quiet the mind, concentrate fully on breathing and counting through each cycle. Repeat this breathing exercise five to ten times and make a habit of doing the exercises several times each day, even when not feeling stressed.

Additional information on deep breathing and stress reduction is available at:

• About.com

  How to Release Tension with Stress Relief Breathing

  http://stress.about.com/od/breathingexercises/ht/breathing-ex.htm

10.2   Cognitive Behavior Therapy

Cognitive behavior is one of the most effective ways to reduce clinically significant stress. This method includes:

• Identifying sources of stress.

  It is useful to start the process of stress reduction with a diary that keeps an informal inventory of daily events and activities. The first step is to note activities that put a strain on energy and time, trigger anger or anxiety, or precipitate a negative physical response (e.g., headache, upset stomach, etc.). Also note positive experiences, such as those that are mentally or physically refreshing or produce a sense of accomplishment and enjoyment. And, after a week or two, try to identify two or three events or activities that have been significantly upsetting or overwhelming.

• Questioning sources of stress.

  One should then question the sources of stress and ask oneself the following questions:

  ▪ do these stressful activities meet my own goals or someone else's?

  ▪ have I taken on tasks that I can reasonably accomplish?

  ▪ which tasks are under my control and which ones aren't?

• Restructuring priorities: adding stress reducing activities.

  The next step is to attempt to shift the balance from stress-producing to stress-reducing activities. Adding daily pleasant events appears to have a more positive effect than reducing negative stressful ones. Also, small daily decisions for improvement accumulate and reconstruct a stressful existence into a more pleasant and productive one. Stress relief options may include such things as:

- if the source of stress is in the home, plan times away, even if it is only an hour or two a week;
- replace unnecessary, time-consuming chores with pleasurable and interesting activities;
- take long weekends/short vacations.

- Keeping perspective and looking for the positive.

  Reversing negative ideas and learning to focus on positive outcomes helps reduce tension/stress and achieve goals. The following steps may be useful:

  - first identify the worst possible outcome;
  - develop a specific plan to achieve the positive outcome;
  - envision a favorable result;
  - rate the likelihood of a bad outcome happening;
  - try to recall previous situations that initially seemed negative but ended well.

- Using humor.

  Keeping a sense of humor during difficult situations is a very effective way to cope with stress. Laughter not only releases tension/stress but also helps keep perspective and reduces stress hormone levels.

- Reducing stress on the job:

  - be sure to schedule daily pleasant activities and physical exercise during free time;
  - establish or reinforce a network of friends at home and at work as well as in your community;
  - learn to focus on positive outcomes;
  - plan and execute a career change if job turns out to be intolerable. Consider transfers within the company;

- restructure priorities and eliminate unnecessary tasks;

- work with Human Resources in a non-confrontational way to improve working conditions, letting them know that productivity can be improved if some of the stress/pressure is off.

• Utilizing various relaxation techniques that prove to be useful.

See Chapter 10 for additional information on relaxation techniques.

10.3   Hypnosis—Self-Hypnosis/Mental Imagery—Visualization

Hypnosis is regarded as an altered state of consciousness. This state of altered consciousness is achieved with the assistance of a hypnotherapist and can be of help not only in relieving stress but also in the therapy of a variety of medical and psychological disorders. Using hypnosis as a therapeutic technique is designed to help one gain control over maladaptive behavior, emotions, and well-being so that stressful situations can be prevented or minimized and one can better cope with the emotional problems and stresses of every day life.

Under the influence of hypnosis, one can learn to be more:

• focused and attentive;

• responsive to suggestions;

• open and less critical and disbelieving in attitude;

• calm, relaxed and less stressed.

Hypnosis "quiets the mind" and enables one to concentrate on a specific thought, memory, feeling or sensation while blocking out distractions. It allows one to be more open to useful suggestions designed to help change harmful attitudes, belief systems, and behaviors thereby improving well-being and health accordingly.

It is important to remember that one does not surrender their free will under hypnosis. Rather, as a hypnotized individual, one is placed in a heightened state of awareness, concentration, and focused attention. In fact one undergoes hypnosis entirely voluntarily. The hypnotherapist only serves as a knowledgeable facilitator or guide.

Generally one does not lose consciousness under hypnosis, or develop amnesia regarding the event. However, a small number of individuals do go into a deep hypnotic state and experience at least some spontaneous amnesia but most remember everything that occurs.

Also, bear in mind that one cannot be put under hypnosis against their will (without their consent). Rather, hypnosis depends on one's willingness to undergo and experience it. And, in fact, not everyone can be hypnotized even with their consent.

Regarding stress reduction/prevention, a variety of hypnotic techniques may be used. The approach chosen depends on the goals and personal preferences of the hypnotherapist and the individual involved in therapy.

The hypnotherapist may lead one into hypnosis in a gentle, soothing voice, describing one or more images that create a sense of well-being, security and relaxation in one who is insecure, anxious, tense, and "stressed out" or drinking, smoking, or eating too much. Under hypnosis, the therapist then suggests ways for the individual in question to achieve specified goals in terms of stress reduction, or smoking or food and alcohol consumption.

Using another approach, the hypnotherapist may stimulate one's imagination by suggesting specific mental images to be visualized. Through such mental imagery/visualization involving the creation of meaningful pictures in one's mind, can prove to be a useful way to enhance one's ability to achieve desired goals.

A third technique is self-hypnosis (auto-suggestion) in which the hypnotherapist teaches one how to induce a state of hypnosis in oneself so that it may be used to reduce stress.

Self-hypnosis is a technique that almost anyone can do daily, allowing one to focus away from thoughts which cause tension/stress. The relaxation exercise described below is a 6 step one derived from Dr. Herbert Benson's book, "The Relaxation Response" as follows:

Step 1—choose a quiet room reasonably free of distraction.

Step 2—sit in a comfortable relaxed position in a cushioned armchair.

Step 3—close both eyes completely.

Step 4—slowly repeat a one syllable word or single digit number silently over and over again for 10–15 minutes.

Step 5—let all that may, happen. When distracting thoughts occur, don't try to analyze them. Rather, disregard them and return to the chosen word or number. Distracting thoughts that occur may indicate release from stress.

Step 6—gradually let yourself come out of the relaxation exercise and sit quietly for a couple of minutes before opening the eyes slowly, enjoying the surroundings and then go about normal daily activities calm, relaxed and alert.

Most individuals feel a sense of well-being after completing the above relaxation exercise. Practice it 2–3 times a day for best results. It can easily be done at home, work or even on vacation. However, it is not advisable to perform this mediation within 2 hours of consuming a meal, alcohol, or medication as these may interfere with results.

Visualization is another excellent tool to deal with stress or dis-ease in life. It is a meditation technique that uses pictures or imagery to "quiet the mind" and return one back to a state of calm and well-being.

The human brain generally is regarded as divided into two sides—the left or logical side and the right or creative side. Most of our lives is spent using the left or logical side, left brain mode for basic survival. However, with visualization, the right or creative side dominates and produces "balance". By yielding to one's right brain, with a positive visualized image, one may access the mind-body connection, restoring balance, and opening up to positive change and healing. Such balance appears to be involved in the natural healing process of the mind-body connection.

When one experiences an emotion in the mind, it produces a feeling that turns into a physical sensation in the body. All one has to do to illustrate this is to remember a sad movie scene that produced tears or a last minute sporting event that produced excitement and enjoyment. Thus visualization of an appropriate image may provide the necessary stimulus that turns into a sensation and changes attitude. This is how one may access the mind-body connection to produce a calming, relaxing sensation to relieve and/or cope with stress.

Remember, one is basically what one thinks—so think positively as often as possible. Negative thoughts/images/visualization keeps one in a more or less unhealthy mental state and may lead to unhealthy bodily function and disease. And negative emotions may delay and prevent one from achieving goals. Positive thinking/visualization may enhance the mind-body connection to work in a more balanced mode which is more conducive to change and healing.

One can learn to live in a more positive, balanced mode by not:
- confusing happiness with fulfillment of desires;
- employing the word "should" too often;
- insisting on being right;
- living in the past or future, and not in the present;
- over controlling situations;
- using rationalization too frequently;
- worrying about what other individuals want.

Remember, by living in the moment, life flows more easily. Through visualization/mental imagery and letting the outcome go, intention can be accomplished—always focusing on the intention and not the result. If the intention is to be stress-free with visualization/imagery—then it is to feel, trust, and know that being stress-free is being accomplished.

Additional information on hypnosis, imagery and visualization is available at:

- About.com

  Hypnosis—What Is It, Who Can Do It

  http://mentalhealth.about.com/cs/specialtechniques/a/hypno.htm

  Using Guided Imagery for Stress Management

  http://stress.about.com/od/generaltechniques/p/profileimagery.htm

- American Psychological Association

  What Is Clinical Hypnosis and What Is It Used for

  http://www.apa.org/releases/hypnosis.html

- Mayo Clinic

  Hypnosis: An Altered State of Consciousness

  http://www.mayoclinic.com/health/hypnosis/SA00084

10.4 Massage Therapy

Massage therapy slows down the heart rate, relaxes the body and reduces stress, at least temporarily. Swedish massage uses muscle manipulation. Shiatsu applies pressure to various parts of the body including the spine. Reflexology manipulates acupressure points in the hands and feet. Although patients appear to prefer therapeutic massage, it is an expensive intervention, requiring significant resources and equipment. On the other hand, relaxation tapes, either used at home or during clinic sessions/doctor's visits, appear to be an equally effective intervention for stress reduction, and much less expensive.

Additional information on massage therapy is available at:

- American Psychological Association

  Get the Massage

  http://www.apa.org/monitor/julaug02/massage.html

- Mayo Clinic

  Massage: A Relaxing Method to Relieve Stress and Pain

  http://www.mayoclinic.com/health/massage/SA00082

10.5   Meditation

Meditation techniques can involve complete stillness or motion. Several different mediation techniques are available including:

- concentration meditation—involves focusing one's attention on a single object like breathing, or an image one visualizes in one's mind such as a lighted candle or a sacred symbol or icon;

- mediation in motion—involves meditation during movement such as walking, yoga or tai chi;

- mediation in prayer—the best known and most widely practiced form of mediation.

Trancendental meditation is a form of concentration meditation and appears to be one of the more popular and useful techniques. TM employs a mantra (a word that has a specific chanting sound but no meaning) to focus on. The meditator repeats the word silently, letting thoughts come and go. A short phrase or prayer may substitute as a mantra.

Meditation appears not only able to reduce stress and stress hormone levels but also decrease blood pressure and heart rate, elevate mood and produce a calming effect.

Additional information on meditation is available at:

- Mayo Clinic

  Meditation: Focusing Your Mind to Achieve Stress Reduction

  http://www.mayoclinic.com/health/meditation/HQ01070

  Tai Chi: Stress Reduction, Balance, Agility and More

  http://www.mayoclinic.com/health/tai-chi/SA00087

  Yoga: Minimize Stress, Maximize Flexibility, and Even More

  http://www.mayoclinic.com/health/yoga/CM00004

- The Transcendental Meditation Program

  Transcendental Meditation ™

  http://www.tm.org

- About.com

  Benefits and Different Types of Mediation

  http://stress.about.com/od/lowstresslifestyle/a/meditation.htm

10.6 Progressive Muscle Relaxation

Progressive muscle relaxation techniques, combined with deep breathing, are simple to learn and useful for relaxation, reducing stress, and inducing sleep in stressed individuals. The technique is carried out as follows.

- lie down in a comfortable position without crossing the limbs, concentrate on each part of the body's muscles;

- maintain a slow, deep breathing pattern throughout this exercise;

- tense each muscle as tightly as possible for a count of five to ten and then release it completely;

- experience the muscle as totally relaxed and "heavy as lead";

- begin with the head and progress downward in the body focusing on all the muscles in the body in sequence from top to bottom;

- be sure to include the forehead, ears, eyes, mouth, neck, shoulders, arms, hands, fingers, chest, abdomen, thighs, calves and feet;

- when the external muscle relaxation is complete, imagine tensing and releasing internal muscles.

Additional information on progressive muscle relaxation and stress reduction is available at:

- Mayo Clinic

  Relax: Techniques to Help You Achieve Tranquility

  http://www.mayoclinic.com/health/relaxation-technique/SR00007

10.7   Tai Chi

Tai chi is a series of gentle movements that can bring about stress reduction, improved flexibility, balance and reduce stress. Sometimes, tai chi is described as "meditation in motion".

To do tai chi, one performs a defined series of postures or movements/exercises in a slow, graceful manner. Each movement or posture flows into the next without pause. It is generally considered safe for individuals of all ages because movements are low impact and put minimal stress on muscles and joints—and thus is appealing to many older adults or those with arthritis or recovering from an injury. Tai chi is reported to offer both physical and mental benefits that may include:

- agility, flexibility, muscle strength, energy and stamina increases;

- feelings of well-being;

- stress reduction.

This may be accompanied by:

- decreased anxiety and depression;

- improved balance and coordination, and decreased number of falls;

- improved sleep quality;

- reduction in blood pressure;

- relief from chronic pain;

- slower bone loss in post-menopausal women.

Additional information on tai chi and stress reduction is available at:

- Mayo Clinic

  Tai Chi: Stress Reduction, Balance, Agility and More

  http://www.mayoclinic.com/health/tai-chi/SA00087

10.8   Yoga

Besides relieving stress and improving the body's flexibility, yoga is reported to help one manage overall health and well-being and cope with certain disorders. The ultimate goal of yoga is to reach complete peacefulness in the body and mind. Traditional practice requires that one adhere to the philosophy of yoga through behavior, diet and meditation to encourage a more flexible, functioning body and a calm mind.

Yoga is part of the Hindu religion and a way of life. It has been around for over 5000 years. There are different forms of yoga. Hatha yoga is the most popular form and focuses on physical poses and controlled breathing.

Yoga is considered to be reasonably safe and reported to offer not only significant stress relief but also other health benefits such as:

- Balance improvement.

  This helps older adults to become steadier on their feet and avoid falls and fractures.

- Increased ability to cope with cancer or other serious disease.

  Individuals and caregivers practicing yoga may improve the quality of their life and sleep better.

- Management of chronic disease.

    Yoga is reported to benefit patients with asthma, cardiovascular disease, carpal tunnel syndrome, memory problems, multiple sclerosis, and osteoarthritis.

Additional information on yoga and stress is available at:

- Mayo Clinic

    Yoga: Minimize Stress, Maximize Flexibility and Even More

    http://www.mayoclinic.com/health/yoga/CM00004

10.9   Spirituality, Stress and Health

Spirituality is a way one may find meaning, hope, comfort, and reduce stress and enjoy inner peace in life. Many individuals find spirituality through organized religion. Others may find it in a connection with nature or their values and principles.

Some research shows that such things as positive beliefs, comfort and inner strength can be gained from religion. And meditation and prayer can contribute to healing and a sense of well-being, and help one better cope with illness, impending death, or the emotional problems of every day living.

Prayer allows communication with our Source (God) in supplication, meditation, appreciation, and application:

- supplication asks for guidance in prayer;
- meditation allows the voice of conscience to be heard;
- appreciation expresses gratitude in grateful, loving thoughts;
- application puts the inner guidance of conscience into action.

As such, prayers help sooth the spirit as one reflects on the meaning and purpose of life.

Prayer is the best known and most widely practiced example of meditation, and is found in most faith traditions. One can pray using one's own words or read prayers written by others either silently or out loud. Read or listened to, one needs to take time to reflect, and focus on one's love, compassion, and gratitude for the many blessings of life.

Everyone prays in their own language and there is no language that God does not understand. Select a prayer technique that fits with your lifestyle and belief system. Set aside some time, 5–20 minutes twice a day, and pray. Keep trying and be kind to yourself as you start. If your mind wanders, slowly return to prayer. Make prayer a part of your life, starting and ending the day with prayer, love, and gratitude.

10.9.1 Centering Prayer

Being present or attentive to another is the foundation of any relationship. And one can think of centering prayer as the cultivation of a personal relationship with God. As such, centering prayer may be described as attentive surrender in silence to God.

Thus, centering prayer is sitting and gazing at a loved one with no need for talking and no agenda. When you pray to God in centering prayer, go into your private room and pray in silence.

Others may be accustomed to vocal or mental prayer or a type of meditation which actively uses the imagination.

10.9.2 Peace Prayer of St. Francis of Assisi

One such well known vocal or mental prayer, is the one attributed to St. Francis of Assisi below:

Lord, make me an instrument of Your Peace!
Where there is hatred, let me sow love;

Where there is injury, pardon;
Where there is error, truth;
Where there is discord, union;
Where there is doubt, faith;
Where there is despair, hope;
Where there is darkness, light;
Where there is sadness, joy.
O' Divine Master,
Grant that I may not so much seek
To be consoled as to console:
To be understood, as to understand;
To be loved, as to love.
For it is in giving that we receive;
It is in pardoning that we are pardoned;
And it is in dying that we are born into eternal life.
Amen.

The peace prayer of St. Frances is a famous prayer which is reported to have first appeared around 1915 AD, and embodies the spirit of St. Francis of Assisi's life of service, simplicity, and poverty. According to Father Kajetan Esser, OPM, the author of the critical edition of St. Francis's writings, the Peace Prayer of St. Francis likely is not one of the writings of St. Francis. The first version of this prayer, apparently appeared during the First World War. It was found written on a holy card of St. Francis which was found in a Norman Almanac. The prayer bore no name, but in the English speaking world, because of this holy card, it came to be called the Prayer of St. Francis.

Different versions of this prayer have appeared since the "original" one, and the one printed in this book is by an unknown author. Nevertheless, I still like to call it the Peace Prayer of St. Francis of Assisi.

10.9.3 The Author's Prayer

My own prayer, which I refer to as The Author's Prayer is given below.

Jesus Christ!
In joyful adoration, profound gratitude, and never-ending praise to Your Splendor and Glory,
I acknowledge and accept You as my Lord and Savior, the Truth, Love, and the Way to peace, happiness, and eternal life.
In loving trust, I surrender my Self, Body, and Soul into Your Hands,
May Your Will be mine and lead me on the path to Everlasting Salvation.
Lord, as I come to You in humility, repentance, and amendment, grant I may be:

> forgiven for my sins
> blessed with Your Amazing Grace
> filled with the Holy Spirit
> transformed and healed in Oneness with You,
> and serve in:
>> love
>> compassion
>> generosity
>> forgiveness
>> mercy, and
>> justice for all

So that I may do my part to help recreate the World according to Your Word.
Amen.

10.9.4   Serenity Prayer

The Serenity Prayer may be found in Chapter 9, Section 9.1.

The Centering Prayer, Peace Prayer of St. Francis of Assisi, Author's Prayer, and Serenity Prayer each have been instrumental in helping the Author cope with the many stresses and emotional problems of everyday living during his life, and are hereby credited accordingly. Hopefully, these prayers will be as helpful to the reader as well.

Remember, "veritas vos liberabit"—the truth will set you free. And, spirituality and prayer can lead one there—to the truth and a much less stressful life and existence.

Additional information on spirituality, stress and health is available at:

- American Family Physician

  Medicine and Society: Providing Basic Spiritual Care for Patients

  http://www.aafp.org/afp/20010101/medicine.html

- Family Doctor

  Spirituality and Health

  http://www.familydoctor.org/650.xml

- Psych Central

  Faith Healing

  http://www.psychcentral.com/psypsch/Spiritual_healing

- About.com

  Achieving Inner Peace and Reducing Stress with Prayer

  http://healing.about.com/od/prayersblessings/a/prayerprocess.htm

- Mayo Clinic

  Meditation: Focusing Your Mind to Achieve Stress Reduction

  http://www.mayoclinic.com/health/meditation/HQ010070

- Duke University

  Duke Spirituality and Health

  http://www.dukespiritualityandhealth.org

  Click on "Research" and go to various reports on the benefits of prayer and religion.

Additional information on St. Francis and the Peace Prayer is available at:

- Catholic.org

  http://www.catholic.org/saints/saint.php?saint_id=50

- Sacred Heart.com

  http://www.thesacredheart.com/pfrantm

- Franciscan Archives

  http://www.franciscan-archive.org/patriacha

Chapter 11 — Searching the Web

Although search engines such as Google and AlltheWeb may provide reasonably complete searches of the Web via their databases, one is left with the very difficult and time consuming task of reviewing the Web pages/reports provided after a search in order to determine which contain current and useful information. Unfortunately, this usually is well beyond the capability of all but a few readers to accomplish satisfactorily in a reasonable period of time.

In order to simplify matters in this regard, the Author has carefully selected, personally reviewed, and assembled the Author's List: Stress Web Resources/Websites in Chapter 12 that are considered to be useful for current stress information. These Web Resources/Websites are listed alphabetically for ease of reference. Each of these Web Resources/Websites provides various stress information reports and/or a Search site and links that may be used to obtain additional information.

This Author's List provides reasonably reliable and useful, up-to-date stress information assembled chiefly by professional organizations, medical schools, or official US governmental resources.

In instituting any search for information using the Author's List, it is important to remember that the Web is growing rapidly, and is in a constant state of flux, updating, and reorganization. Web Resources listed may change/modify their name and/or website address, format, content and categorization/display of information, as well as delete or change Web pages/reports.

If for any reason, one finds that the Website chosen doesn't produce the information one is seeking, search the Web Resource name, report or subject itself. Should a problem still persist, try another search engine to access the Web resource name, Website, report, or subject in question.

Web Resources use different methods to search the Web to compile their database. Each Web Resource organizes/assembles information differently, some better than others. Thus, different Web resources/Websites likely will provide information that may differ significantly and need to be reconciled. And, Web pages/reports/information may be changed or removed or temporarily become unavailable on any given Web Resource/Website for a number of reasons.

In general, stress and stress-management information obtained via the Author's List may be regarded as reasonably current and useful in most instances/respects but not necessarily all. Unlike medical/scientific articles published in peer review journals, there is no guarantee that information obtained from any single Web Resource/Website in the Author's list may necessarily be relied upon in its entirety as the "gospel truth". Therefore, information from a minimum of at least two to three other Web Resources/Websites needs to be compared and reconciled, when different. Also, in the amazing world of the Web, a second, or even a third, opinion is considered to be worthwhile.

Even in the world of scientific evidence-based information from well-controlled trials, there may be problems in terms of what the data collected and results may mean. Clinical trial evidence necessarily is subject to interpretation and application, both subjective processes.

Everyone is biased to some degree in one way or another in obtaining, analyzing, interpreting and applying information, evidence-based or not. Words, phrases, statistics, and conclusions mean different things to different people at different times and places depending on "where one is coming from" so to speak. For example, even in the case of the Constitution of the United States of America, written by "great minds", individuals, lawyers, judges, congressmen and senators, and even the Supreme Court of the United States still continue to argue, debate, disagree about, and usually have great difficulty in interpreting and applying the so-called "original intent" of the "founding fathers" of this great document.

Nevertheless, one may entertain a reasonable degree of confidence that the stress and stress management information obtained via the Web resources/Websites cited in this book may help one become better informed in order to understand and cope with stress and live a healthier, happier, longer and more productive life.

Chapter 12 — Author's List:
Stress Web Resources/Websites

12.1   About.com/a New York Times Company

http://www.about.com/stress

About.com is a company acquired in 2006 by the New York Times and visited by around 30 million people each month. Their "Guides" are reported to offer practical advice and possible solutions for everyday life, including stress. According to Nielsen Net Ratings, About.com is a top 10 Web property used by one out of every five people on the Internet. Featured stress sites/reports include:

- *Stress Basics: Types of Stress and Your Health and How Stress Works*

  http://stress.about.com/od/understandingstress/a/stress_basics.htm

  The first step in conquering stress is understanding the basics of stress.

- *Stress Management Site*

  http://stress.about.com/index.htm

  Learn about the causes and effects of stress, healthy and effective coping strategies, time management and organization tips. Find support and information for stressed parents, workers, students, and others who would like to experience less stress and enjoy life more.

- *Stress and Health: How Stress Affects Your Body, Stress and Health Conditions, and How You Can Stay Healthier*

  http://stress.about.com/stresshealth/a/stresshealth.htm

- *Top Ten Stress Relievers: The Best Ways to Feel Better*

  http://stress.about.com/od/generaltechniques/tp/toptensionacts.htm

  There are many ways to reduce stress. Here are ten stress relievers that are regarded as reasonably effective.

- *Financial Stress: Managing Your Money—and Your Stress*

  http://stress.about.com/od/financialstress

- *Financial Tools for Stress Reduction*

  http://stress.about.com/od/financialtools

- *Financial Stress: How it Affects You and What You Can Do*

  http://stress.about.com/financialstress/financialstress.htm

- *Relaxation*

  http://stress.about.com/cs/relaxation/index.htm

  Relaxation techniques including biofeedback, stress management, breathing control, imagery, mediation, yoga, hypnosis, progressive muscle relaxation and more.

  Hypnosis—What Is It, Who Can Do It

  http://mentalhealth.about.com/cs/specialtechniques/a/hypno.htm

  How to Release Tension with Stress Relief Breathing

  http://stress.about.com/od/breathingexercises/ht/breathing-ex.htm

- *What Stresses You the Most*

  http://stress.about.com/library/polls/blstresspoll1.htm

12.2   American Academy of Family Physicians (AAFP)

http://www.aafp.org

AAFP is one of the largest national medical organizations, representing more than 94,000 family medicine healthcare providers nationwide. Founded in 1947, its mission has been to preserve and promote the science and art of family medicine and to ensure high-quality, cost-effective healthcare for patients of all ages.

Links/reports on "anger" and "stress" can be found via the Search site on the AAFP website, including the following reports:

<u>Anger</u>

- *Conference Highlight: Anger*
  http://www.aafp.org/afp/980600ap/conhigh.html
- *Mental Health: Keeping Your Emotional Health*
  http://www.aafp.org/aafp/20021001/1287ph.html
- *Curbside Consultation: Understanding Anger in Parents of Dying Children*
  http://www.aafp.org/afp/981001ap/consult.html
- *Grieving: Facing Illness, Death and Other Loses*
  http://familydoctor.org/079.xml
- *Identifying and Managing Preparatory Grief and Depression at the End of Life*
  http://www.aafp.org/afp/20020301/883.pdf
- *Depression in Women: Diagnostic and Treatment Considerations*
  http://www.aafp.org/afp/990700ap/225.html
- *Tension Type Headache*
  http://www.aafp.org/afp/20020901/797.html
- *Becoming Parents: What It Means for Couples*
  http://www.familydoctor.org/843.xml
- *Depression in Later Life*
  http://www.aafp.org/afp/20040515/2375.html

<u>Stress</u>

- *Ideas for Managing Stress and Extinguishing Burnout*
  http://www.aafp.org/fpm/20020400/35eigh.html
- *Managing Stress from the Inside Out*
  http://www.aafp.org/fpm/20050500/102mana.html
- *Diagnosis and Management of Post-Traumatic Stress Disorder*
  http://www.aafp/org/afp/20031215/2401.html
- *Does Therapeutic Massage Effectively Relieve Stress?*
  http://www.aafp/org/afp/20030601/tips/7.html

12.3   American College of Preventive Medicine (ACPM)

http://www.acpm.org

ACPM is the national professional society for physicians committed to disease prevention and health promotion. Some 2,000 or so members are engaged in preventive medicine practice, teaching and research. Many serve on ACPM committees and task forces, and represent preventive medicine in national forums, contributing to the organization's role as a major national resource of expertise in disease prevention and health promotion. Specialist members in preventive medicine are uniquely trained in both clinical medicine and public health. They have the skills needed to understand and reduce the risks of disease, disability and death in individuals and population groups. ACPM physicians can be found in primary care, managed care organizations, public health and government agencies, and in industry and academia. ACPM provides useful information on the mind/body connection—how emotions affect your health.

Individuals with emotional health are aware of their thoughts, feelings and behaviors and have learned healthy ways to cope with the stress and problems of every day living, a normal aspect of life. Healthy people feel satisfied with themselves and have good relationships and low stress lifestyles.

However, many events in life can disrupt emotional health—leading to stress, anxiety and/or depression. These events may include such things as being laid off from work, having a child leave or return home, serious illness, death of a family member or a loved one, divorce, money problems, relocating or having a baby.

Our body responds to the way one thinks, feels, or acts via the mind/body connection. Under stress, the body tells you in various ways that all is not well. For example, high blood pressure, a stroke, an acute coronary event, or a stomach upset may present as problems/disorders indicating that one's emotional health is out of balance and "stressed out".

Stress can weaken one's body in many ways. Also, when one is feeling stressed, anxious, or depressed one may not take care of one's health as well as one should.

ACPM site provides much useful information for preventing, recognizing and coping with stress via their Search site. "Stress" and "stress management", information provided includes:

- self management: taking charge of one's health;
- what is self management of chronic illness and how can it help;
- what can I do to keep myself healthy;
- what preventive services do all adults need;
- what preventive services do men need;
- what preventive services do women need;
- healthy living: how common behaviors affect your health;
- what are the most common causes of death and what can I do to reduce my risk;

- mind/body connection: how emotions affect health. What is good emotional health.

12.4   American Institute of Stress (AIS)

http://www.stress.org

AIS is dedicated to advancing the understanding of the role of stress in health and illness, the nature and importance of mind-body relationships, and our inherent and immense potential for self-healing.

AIS regards stress as "America's #1 Health Problem" and job stress as the "major culprit". Click on the home page to find out more about stress.

Stress is regarded by AIS as an unavoidable consequence of life. As Hans Selye (who coined the term stress as it is currently used) noted: "Without stress, there would be no life". AIS states that "just as distress can cause disease, it seems plausible that there are good stresses that promote wellness. Stress is not always necessarily harmful. Winning a race or an election can be just as stressful as losing, or more so, but may trigger a very different biological response. Increased stress results in increased productivity—up to a point. However, this level differs for each of us. It is very much like stress on a violin string. Not enough produces a dull raspy sound. Too much tension makes a shrill, annoying noise or snaps the string. However, just the right degree can create a magnificent tone. Similarly, we all need to find the proper level of stress that allows us to perform optimally and make melodious music as we go through life".

AIS is committed to developing a better understanding of how to tap into the vast potential that resides in each of us for preventing disease and promoting good health which is more than the absence of illness. Good health is a very robust state of physical and emotional well-being, which acknowledges the importance and inseparability of mind/body relationships. In this regard, it is important to remember:

"Always fight for your highest attainable aim but never put up resistance in vain."

Hans Selye

September, 2005 marked the launch of the American Psychological Association (APA) Mind/Body Health Campaign to educate people across the USA that when it comes to your body, your mind really matters, and that focusing on the unhealthy behaviors behind poor physical heath is as important as focusing on the physical symptoms.

AIS is one of the cooperating organizations for the campaign. The APA Help Center website—http://www.apahelpcenter.org—is full of information about the Mind/Body connection that one may find helpful via click on key links/reports, namely:

- *Mind/Body Health: Did You Know*
- *Mind/Body Health: Job Stress*
- *Mind/Body Health: Heart Disease*
- *Mind/Body Health: Obesity*

AIS special reports are also available via click on links for the following key reports:

- *Stress and Hypertension*—an interview with Dr. John Laragh by Paul J. Rosch, M.D., F.A.C.P., the American Institute of Stress

- *Type A and Coronary Disease*—separating fact from fiction, an interview by Dr. Ray Rosenman

- *Speaking Heart to Heart*—an interview with Dr. James T. Lynch, author of "The Broken Heart: the Medical Consequences of Loneliness", "The Language of the Heart". "A Cry Unheard", and "Speaking of Love".

12.5   American Psychiatric Association (APA)

http://www.psych.org

The American Psychiatric Association (APA) is recognized world-wide as a premier mental health organization composed primarily of psychiatrists. Its over 36,000 U.S. and international member physicians work together to ensure humane and effective treatment for all persons with mental disorders, mental retardation, substance abuse disorders, and stress-related mental health problems.

The APA search site is serviced by Google. Click-on websites/reports are made available via a search of "stress" and "stress management".

A number of recent book references also are featured. Among these are:

- *Fear and Anxiety*, 2004

  Edited by: Jack M. Gorman

- *Treatment of Stress Response Syndromes*, 2003

  Mardi J. Horowitz, M.D.

- *What Every Patient, Family, Friend and Caregiver Needs to Know About Psychiatry*, 2nd Edition, 2003

  Richard W. Roukema, M.D., F.A.P.A.

- *Stress, Mental Disorders, and Health*, 2000

  Edited by Karl Goodkin, M.D., Ph.D. and Adrian P. Visser, M.D

- *Nature and Nurture in Psychiatry: A Predisposition—Stress Model of Mental Disorders*, 1999

  Joel Paris, M.D.

- *Does Stress Cause Psychiatric Illness*, 1994

  Edited by: Carolyn M. Mazure, Ph.D.

- *Post-traumatic Stress Disorder*, 1993

  Edited by: R.T. Davidson, M.D. and Edna B. Foa, Ph.D.

12.6   American Psychological Association (APA)

http://www.apa.org

The American Psychological Association (APA) is a scientific and professional organization that represents psychology. With around 150,000 members, APA is the largest association of psychologists worldwide.

Psychology is the study of the mind and behavior, and the discipline embraces all aspects of the human experience—from the functions of the brain to the actions of nations, and from child developments to care of the aged. In every conceivable setting from scientific research centers to mental health care services, "the understanding of behavior" is regarded as the enterprise of psychologists.

There are 53 professional divisions in the APA. This website also contains the list of the divisions organized by topic area. These can be found at: http://www.apa.org/about/division.html

A search of "stress" at the APA website provides click-on websites/reports for information on stress. Some of these click-on sites/reports include:

- *Stress: Information for the Public*

  Additional information for the public on stress

- *Hard Hitting Hormones: The Stress-Depression Link*

  Chronic stress has long been shown to fuel depression.

- *Mental Stress May be Another Culprit in Raising Cholesterol Levels in Healthy Adults: Increases Risk for Heart Problems*

  Stress increases the risk of CVD.

- *Stress Affects Immunity in Ways Related to Type and Duration*

  As shown by nearly 300 studies

- *Post-traumatic Stress Disorder (PTSD)*

  A primer on PTSD

- *Couples Coping With Stress*

  How couples cope with acute and chronic stress, within and outside the family.

- *Elder Abuse and Neglect: In Search of Solutions*

  Covers different types of elder abuse and neglect and why such abuse occurs.

- *Money Issues: Leading Cause of Holiday Stress for Americans*

  Money issues constitute top vote getters for holiday stress according to a recent APA poll.

- *Preventive Stress Management in Organizations*

  Provides orderly framework for practicing healthy preventive stress management.

- *What's to Blame for the Surge in Super-Size Americans*

  Discusses the environmental, biological, and genetic factors cited by some of the nation's top obesity experts that make losing and even maintaining, weight an uphill battle, and lists some possible solutions.

- *Turning Lemons into Lemonade: Hardiness Helps People Turn Stressful Circumstances into Opportunities*

  Hardiness is the key to the resiliency needed not only to survive but to thrive under stress.

- *Road, Rage, Air Rage and Now "Desk" Rage*

  Work stress is leading more people to engage in counter productive work place behaviors.

- *Experts Testify on the Importance of Stress Management in Fighting Heart Disease*

  Summary of 37 studies shows that stress management and lifestyle change programs can help reduce the number of deaths from heart disease by 34 percent.

In searching the topic "anger" at the APA site, the following click on sites/reports are available:

- abuse and anger fixation
- advances in anger management
- anger on the road
- controlling anger before it controls you
- managing anger
- warning signs: controlling you own risk for violent behavior
- warning signs: dealing with anger
- when anger is a plus

Regarding the topic "anxiety", the following sites/reports are available via the APA search site:

- cognitive behavioral treatment
- conquering fear
- fighting phobias
- knowledge perspective can lessen terrorism-anxiety
- new approach to complicated grief
- new data shed light on anxiety
- normal responses to abnormal situations
- second guessing jeopardizes mental health

Concerning "depression", the following sites/reports are available:

- depression and how psychotherapy and other treatments can help people recover
- exercise helps keep your psyche fit
- facts about depression in older adults
- family financial woes can foster child depression and disobedience

- happiness and self esteem: can one exist without the other
- marital satisfaction affected by both spouses mental health
- memory accentuates the positive, helping explain why aging can foster good feelings
- poorer people with depression are harder to treat
- probing the puzzling workings of depressive realism
- unhappiness has risen in the past decade

12.7   Family Doctor (FD)

http://www.familydoctor.org

FD is operated by the Academy of Family Physicians (AAFP), a national medical organization representing about 90,000 family physicians devoted to family medicine/care. All of the information on this site has been written and reviewed by physicians and education professionals at the AAFP.

Searching for "stress" provides click on sites/reports on stress information graded by stars, from 1–4, indicating the degree of relevance to the search. The higher the number of stars, the greater the relevance.

Reports provided with two or more stars include:
- *Stress: Who Has Time for It?* (4 stars)
  http://www.familydoctor.org/278.xml
- *Stress: How to Cope Better with Life's Challenges* (4 stars)
  http://www.familydoctor.org/167.xml
- *Caregiver Stress* (3 stars)
  http://www.familydoctor.org.645.xml
- *Mind/Body Connection* (3 stars)
  http://www.familydoctor.org/782.xml

- *Post-traumatic Stress After a Traffic Accident* (2 stars)

  http://www.familydoctor.org/449.xml

- *Sexual Dysfunction in Women: What Can I Do If Sex Isn't Working for Me?* (2 stars)

  http://www.familydoctor.org/612.xml

- *Irritable Bowel Syndrome: Tips on Controlling Your Symptoms* (2 stars)

  http://www.familydoctor.org/112.xml

- *Cancer: When You're a Caregiver* (2 stars)

  http://www.familydoctor.org/719.xml

- *Healthy Living* (2 stars)

  http://www.familydoctor.org/healthy.xml

- *High Blood Pressure: Things You Can Do to Help Lower Yours* (2 stars)

  http://www.familydoctor.org/092.xml

- *Smoking: Don't Let It Steer You Wrong* (2 stars)

  http://www.familydoctor.org274.xml

- *Weight Control: Choosing the Right Diet to Lose Weight* (2 stars)

  http://www.familydoctor.org/796.xml

- *Migraine Headache: Ways to Deal with Pain* (2 stars)

  http://www.familydoctor.org/127.xml

- *Erectile Dysfunction* (2 stars)

  http://www.familydoctor.org/109.xml

- *Tension Headache* (2 stars)

  http://www.familydoctor.org/172.xml

12.8   HealthFinder (HF)

http://www.healthfinder.gov

HF is a service of the National Health Information Center, U.S. Department of Health and Human Services. It has been recognized since 1997 as a key resource for finding the best government and non-profit health and human services information on the Internet. HF links to carefully selected information from over 1,500 health-related organizations.

The HF project is coordinated by the Office of Disease Prevention and Health Promotion (ODPHP) and its National Health Information Center with the active participation of a Steering Committee composed of representatives of the Federal agencies who include consumer health information specialists, librarians, and others actively engaged in the provision or use of online consumer health information. It is non-profit and supported solely by U.S. Government funds and does not accept paid advertisements, content, or links in any form.

HF is regarded as one of the Medical Library Association's "Top Ten" Most Useful Websites. This website provides much useful information on stress, stress management and stress-related disease.

Included are the following click-on sites/reports:

- *Post-Traumatic Stress Disorder*

  An anxiety disorder that can develop after exposure to a terrifying event or ordeal in which grave physical/psychological harm occurred or was threatened.

- *Stress: Learn What Stress Is and How to Cope*
  ABCs of stress.

- *After a Disaster: Self-Care Tips for Dealing with Stress*
  Ways to ease stress.

- *Healthy Aging: the 40s—Middle-Aged, Mega-Stressed*

  Simple steps can help you cope with everyday anxiety.

- *Holiday Stress*

  Tips on how to cope with holiday stress.

- *Systemic Stress Management*

  Structured program designed to prevent and minimize the damaging effects of stress.

- *Caregiving: Managing the Stress of Care Giving*

  Discusses coping skills that have helped others deal with related issues.

- *Crises Fact Sheet: 5 Ways to Cope with Crisis*

  Fact sheet written by the American Counseling Association recommends 5 ways to cope with a crisis situation.

- *Mind/Body Connection: How Your Emotion Affects Your Health*

  Your body responds to the way you think, feel and act. This is called the "mind/body connection". When you are stressed, anxious or upset, your body tries to tell you that something is not right.

- *Risk Factors for Heart and Blood Vessel Disease*

  Presents risk factors for heart and blood vessel disease and what one can do about them. Risk factors include high blood pressure, smoking, diabetes, stress, and family history.

12.9   Mayo Clinic (MC)

http://www.mayoclinic.com

The mission of the Mayo Clinic is to empower people to manage their health. This is accomplished by providing useful, up-to-date information and tools that reflect the expertise and standard of excellence of the Mayo Clinic.

A team of Web-publishing professionals and medical experts produce this site. Through this unique collaboration, you are provided with access to the experience and knowledge of more than 2,000 physicians and scientists of the Mayo Clinic and the Mayo Foundation for Medical Education.

A search of "stress" and "anger" on the MC site provides a number of click-on links/reports which include the following:

- *Massage: A Relaxing Method to Relieve Stress and Pain*

  http://www.mayoclinic.com/health/massage/SA00082

- *Stress Center*

  http://www.mayoclinic.com/heath/stress/SR99999

  Practical and credible stress management strategies for stress reduction/relief.

- *Stress: Why You Have It and How It Hurts Your Health*

  http://www.mayoclinic.com/health/stress/SR00001

  Constant stress can increase your cholesterol and blood pressure, etc. as well as suppress your immune system and cause an upset stomach.

- *Stress, Depression and the Holidays: 12 Tips for Coping*

  http://www.mayoclinic.com/health/stress/MH00030

  Key ways to cope with holiday stress and depression.

- *Meditation: Focusing Your Mind to Achieve Stress Reduction*

  http://www.mayoclinic.com/health/meditation/HQ01070

  Try meditation for stress reduction.

- *Tai Chi: Stress Reduction, Balance, Agility and More*

  http://www.mayoclinic.com/health/tai-chi/SA00087

  Achieve stress reduction, relaxation and increased flexibility.

- *Yoga: Minimize Stress, Maximize Flexibility and Even More*

  http://www.mayoclinic.com/health/yoga/CM00004

  A popular means of stress reduction, relaxation and increased flexibility.

- *Positive Thinking: A Skill for Stress Relief*

  http://www.mayoclinic.com/health/positive-thinking/SR0009

  Stress management requires positive perspective—knowing how to turn pessimism into optimism.

- *Anger Management: How Angry Are You?*

  http://www.mayoclinic.com/health/anger-management/MH00073

  It is natural to get angry but it isn't healthy to explode—rank your anger.

- *Anger Management: Tips to Control Your Temper*

  http://www.mayoclinic.com/health/anger-managemnt/MH00102

  It is not always bad when controlled. Get tips on anger management.

- *Resilience: Build Skills to Endure Hardship*

  http://www.mayoclinic.com/health/resilience/MH00078

  Improve your resilience so that you can handle life's hardships better.

- *Work-life Balance: Ways to Restore Harmony and Reduce Stress*

  http://www.mayoclinic.com/work-lifebalance/WL00056

  When your work-life and personal-life are out of balance, your stress level can soar. Find out how to restore harmony.

- *Caregiving: Maintain Your Support Network*

  http://www.mayoclinic.com/health/alzheimers-caregiver/AZ00018

- *Long Term Care for Your Parents: What to Consider*

  http://www.mayoclinic.com/health/long-term-care/HQ01517

- *Job Burnout: Don't Let a Demanding Job Affect Your Health*
  http://www.mayoclinic.com/health/burnout/WL00062
  Find out who is prone and what can be done about it.
- *Getting Along with Your Supervisor: When Styles Collide*
  http://www.mayoclinic.com/health/stress/WL00049
  Getting along well with your supervisor increases your job satisfaction and lowers stress. Learn how to make the most of this key relationship.
- *Effective Time Management: Build Your Organizational Skills*
  http://www.mayoclinic.com/health/time-management/WL00048
  Manage your time and reduce stress.

A search of "Stress Center" provides links/reports for additional information/reports on:

- *Signs and Symptoms of Stress: Prompt Recognition is Crucial*
  http://www.mayoclinic.com/health/stress-symptoms/SR00008_D
- *Family Therapy: Healing Family Conflicts*
  http://www.mayoclinic.com/health/family-therapy/HQ00662
- *Hypnosis: An Altered State of Consciousness*
  http://www.mayoclinic.com/health/hypnosis/SA00084
- *Workplace Stress Self-assessment*
  http://www.mayoclinic.com/health/stress/WL00064

12.10 MedicineNet (MN)

http://www.medicinenet.com

MedicineNet (MN) is an online, healthcare media publishing company. It provides easy-to-read, in depth, authoritative medical information for consumers. Since 1996, MN has had an accomplished, experienced network of over 70 US board certified physicians providing you with a trusted source for online health information.

On the home page of MN, under "Should You Know These Conditions", click on the link for "Stress" for reports concerning:

- *What is stress*
- *Brief history of stress*
- *What is the healthy response to stress*
- *How does the response to stress work*
- *Conclusions about the effects of stress*
- *How can we manage stress*
- *What's in the future for stress*

12.11 MedlinePlus (MP)

http://www.medlineplus.gov

Medlineplus brings together authoritative information from the National Library of Medicine (NLM), the National Institutes of Health (NIH), and other government agencies, and health-related organizations. Pre-formulated MEDLINE searches are included in MedlinePlus and give easy access to medical journal articles. MedlinePlus also has extensive information about drugs, an illustrated medical encyclopedia, interactive patient tutorials, and latest health news. MP provides information from over 17,000 links to authoritative health information from over 1,250 organizations.

Searching "stress" and "stress management" on the MP site, click-on sites/reports can be found for:

- backaches and stress
- childhood stress
- coping with disasters

- heart attack

- manage your stress: ten ways to ease stress

- managing traumatic stress: tips for recovering

- Mom's stress impacts her view of child's behavior

- news on new stress research findings

- parents keys to how to handle stress

- stress ABCs

- stress management

Searching "anger" and "anger management" on the MP site, click on sites/reports maybe found for:

- aggressive behavior

- anger

- anger management: how angry are you?

- caring for relatives with a mental disorder

- child behavior disorder

- chronic pain: managing your emotions

- discipline

- maintaining your own health: for family members

- managing stress and recovering from trauma: facts and resources for veterans and families, how do people respond during traumatic exposure?

- managing violence

- mental health: keeping your emotional health

- parents: be models for your children

- teen violence

- understanding violent behavior in children and adolescents

12.12 Mental Help Net (MHN)

http://www.mentalhelp.net

Mental Help Net is an established, highly regarded internet website dedicated to educating its public about mental health, wellness, and family and relationship issues and concerns. It is the recipient of many awards and citations, including being selected as the "Forbes Favorite" mental health website. Designed and maintained by clinical psychologists since it first launched in November 1995, the site provides useful and up-to-date information while maintaining an independent editorial stance. News, articles, reviewed links, interactive tests, book reviews, self-help resources, therapist listing, and even videos make up the varied content to be found in MHN's many topic centers.

MHN is a public service of CenterSite, LLC, an Ohio based provider of high quality, affordable website services to employee assistance programs, substance abuse centers and community health centers.

A click on list of mental disorders, a brief discussion of each, featured symptoms and treatment as well as organizations concerned is provided.

Additional information, is made available under Detailed Information, News, Videos, Links, Book Reviews, and Self-Help Groups, etc.

Searching information for "stress" via the MHN Search site provides click-on links/reports including:

- *Stress Could Shrink the Brain*

  New research indicates that stress does more than just cause a headache—it may actually damage the hippocampus responsible for complex memory.

- *Emotional Resilience*

  Collection of skills, characteristics, habits and outlooks that make it possible to remain maximally flexible and fresh in the face of stress.

- *Environmental Causes: Stress/Depression Primer*

  Does stress cause depression or does depression cause stress?

- *Stress Reduction*

  ➤ learning to achieve the right balance of stress

  ➤ unhealthy methods of coping with stress include: addictions to alcohol, drugs, sex, or gambling.

  ➤ positive, healthy ways include: relaxation/meditation, exercise, healthy/prudent diet, socialization/supportive conversation, assertive communication, time management, and asking for assistance

- *Understanding Pathological Grief*

  Handling grief and bereavement issues

- *Stress and Women's Health*

  With all going on in a woman's life, it is important to find ways to de-stress—your health depends on it.

- *Stress in Middle-Age Ups Diabetes Risk*

  Psychological stress caused by such things as the death of a spouse, a financial crisis, or other life-altering event may increase the risk of developing diabetes.

- *Does Your Morning Coffee Make You Stressed?*

  People who drink four or five cups of coffee through the morning have elevated blood pressure and higher levels of stress hormones all day and into the evening—and the body may act like it is continually under stress.

- *Stress: It's Not All in Your Head*

  Feeling stressed out also shows up in our bodies—cardiovascular disease, diabetes, etc. Exercise, prudent diet, healthy lifestyle appear to be the best antidotes.

- *Psychological Consequences of Being Overweight*

  Psychological consequences of being overweight or obese may include lowered self-esteem and anxiety, or more serious disorders such as distress, depression and eating disorders such as binge eating, bulimia and anorexia.

- *Overworked Couple Have Worst Quality Stress*

  These couples tend to experience more conflict (stress) between work and personal life, more stress and more feelings of overload as well as lack of control and mastery of their lives than others.

- *How to Practice Safe Stress: Interview with "The Stress Doc"*

  Yes, according to the Stress Doc—Mark Gorkin, there is good or eustress, the optimal level of mind/body activation and alertness that facilitates performance. Create some activity in your life for which you have a sense of purpose and passion (and try adding a little playfulness, as well). Mix in disciplined practice and patience and you too will experience the fulfilling glow and gold glow of "good stress".

- *Health Costs of Anger*

  Anger is both a physiological (body) and psychological (mind) process and can have a negative impact on your physical and emotional health. This is particularly true of the relationship between anger and cardiovascular disease.

- *Maintaining Gains: Preparing for Relapse: Smoking Cessation*

  The planning stage doesn't end after you've smoked your last cigarette, etc. To remain smoke free, plan ahead and formulate strategies to deal with temptations. Provides strategies you might consider.

- *A Primer on Coping (and Some Holiday Applications)*

  Within a range of possible ways to cope with a stressor, some are reasonable and might be expected to work (e.g. talking, walking away for a short while, etc.) while others probably won't work as well to resolve a conflict (worrying, yelling, denying or distracting one's self, etc.).

- *The Art and Application of Healing Humor*

  As that great humanitarian and undaunted perceptual pioneer, Helen Keller, observed: "The world is so full of care and sorrow that it is a gracious debt we owe to one another to discover the bright crystals of light hidden in somber circumstances and irksome tasks" from Mark Gorkin, LICSW, "The Stress Doc".

- *How Resilience Works*

  ➤ The attitudes that underlie emotional resilience are powerful because they enable people who subscribe to them to cope with great efficiency and effectiveness.

  ➤ Stress is stressful precisely because it is a source of negative emotions: depression, anxiety, and anger that exert a powerful influence over perception.

  ➤ Rational challenging of negatively exaggerated perceptions is another effective method for lifting one's mood.

- *Transitioning Into Care*

  The start of care, in whatever form that care will take, requires that the elder adjust to being cared for. Because the transition into care is stressful, it is helpful that it occur in stages, over a period of several years, rather than all at once. Breaking the transition into stages makes it possible to break the stress associated with stress care into more manageable chunks.

Anger is a basic human emotion that is experienced by all people at one time or another. It is typically triggered by an emotional hurt and is experienced as an unpleasant feeling when one believes that they have been injured, mistreated or opposed in long held views—or when one is faced with obstacles that do not allow attaining a personal goal. Anger styles are learned and become chronic and a way of life leading to great personal health and social costs. Mental Help Net provides a useful overview of information on anger as follows:

- Introduction

- What is anger
- Psychology of anger
- Anger styles are learned
- Motivational effects of anger
- Health costs of anger
- Societal costs of anger
- Deciding to manage anger
- Recognizing anger signs
- Rage ratings
- Anger diary and triggers
- Relaxation techniques
- Reality testing
- Believable reasons for staying cool
- Assertive communication
- Anger management programs
- Anger contracting
- Handling relapse

To obtain the aforementioned anger information, use the MHN search site: inset the term "anger" and then click on "Docs" and "go". On the first page of resources shown, scroll down and click on "Introduction" and begin reading. Click on the next topic at the bottom of each page to advance to the next in order to read all anger topics.

Note: All MHN information provided is for educational purposes only and not intended to be a substitute for any professional medical advice, diagnosis, or treatment. Always seek the advice of your physician or other qualified health provider with any questions you may have regarding a medical condition.

12.13 Mind Body Medical Institute (MBMI)

http://www.mbmi.org

The Mind Body Medical Institute is regarded as a world leader in the study, advancement and clinical practice of mind/body medicine. Herbert Benson, M.D., is President of MBMI and is a Professor of Medicine at Harvard Medical School.

At the MBMI's newly updated site, you can find useful, up-to-date information on mind/body medicine and stress, as well as help if you are experiencing the negative effects of stress and you can learn how to elicit the relaxation response.

Via the MBMI Search site, numerous click-on sites/reports are made available including the following:

*   *What is Stress*

    http://www.mbmi.org/basics/whatis_stress.asp
*   *Managing Stress*

    http://www.mbmi.org/basics/mstress.asp
*   *Combat Job Stress*

    http://www.mbmi.org/basics/mstress_CJS.asp
*   *Program Teaches Students to Manage Stress*

    http://www.mbmi.org/about/articles/press/teaching_students.pdf
*   *Fertility Improves When Stress is Set Aside*

    http://www.mbmi.org/about/articles/press/relax_fertility.pdf
*   *MBMI—38 Stress Busters*

    http://www.mbmi.org/basics/mstress_SB.asp
*   *The Stress Response*

    http://www.mbmi.org/basics/whatis_stress_response.asp

- *The Relaxation Response*

  http://www.mbmi.org/basics/whatis_rresponse.asp

- *Staying Healthy in a Stressful World*

  http://www.mbmi.org/about/articles/press/staying_healthy2.pdf

- *Mind/Body Practices Help Couples Regain Control*

  http://www.mbmi.org/about/articles/press/infertility_couples.pdf

- *Relieving Holiday Stress*

  http://www.mbmi.org/programs/wellness_holiday.asp

- *Positive Thinking*

  http://www.mbmi.org/basics/whatis_pthinking.asp

- *Especially for Women*

  http://www.mbmi.org/programs/forwomen.asp

- *What is Mind/Body Medicine*

  http://www.mbmi.org/basics/whatis.asp

- *Meditation*

  http://www.mbmi.org/about/articles/press/businessweek.pdf

"Mind/Body medicine can lead you to become more involved in your healthcare and to make positive changes in your life. Health is not simply the absence of illness", from the Wellness Book by Herbert Benson, M.D.

12.14 National Institute for Occupational Safety and Health (NIOSH)

http://www.cdc.gov/niosh/homepage.html

NIOSH is the federal agency responsible for conducting research and making recommendations for the prevention of work-related injuries and illness. NIOSH is part of the Centers for Disease Control and Prevention (CDC) in the Department of Health and Human Services.

The Board of Scientific Counselors of NIOSH is composed of renowned scientists from a variety of fields related to occupational safety and health. They provide advice and guidance in developing and evaluating research, systematically documenting findings, and disseminating results designed to improve the safety and health of workers.

Primary themes in the NIOSH job stress program are to:

1. better understand the influence of what are commonly termed "work organization" or "psychosocial" factors on job stress, illness and injury, and

2. to identify ways to redesign jobs to create safer and healthier workplaces.

In 1996, NIOSH established an interdisciplinary team of researchers and practitioners from industry, labor, and academia to develop a national research agenda on the organization of work. This refers to management and supervisory practices to production processes, and their influence on the way work is performed as a collaborative effort by NIOSH and National Occupational Research Agenda (NORA)—to guide occupational safety and health research into the next decade.

NIOSH also plays an active role in promoting the new field of occupation health psychology (OHP). Many psychologists have argued that the psychology field needs to take a more active role in research and practice to prevent occupational stress, illness, and injury. This is what the new field of OHP is all about. NIOSH feels strongly that OHP should give special attention to the primary prevention of organizational risk factors for stress, illness, and injury at work—that OHP concerns itself with the application of psychology to improve the quality of work life, and to protect and promote the safety, health, and well-being of workers.

Searching "stress" on the NIOSH search site provides a number of click-on sites/reports including:

- *Stress* (NIOSH/DHHS Publication No. 99-101)

  Web pages on stress

  ➢ occupational health psychology

  ➢ quality of work life questionnaire

  ➢ work stress publications

- NIOSH books and videos about stress

  ➢ *Working With Stress*—video

    A brief introduction to work stress issues for the worker and manager. Topics include the causes of job stress, physical and psychological effects, and what can be done to minimize job stress. The video is available on both DVD and VHS formats and can also be viewed online (17 minutes).

  ➢ *Stress At Work*—booklet

    This booklet highlights knowledge about the causes of stress at work and outlines steps that can be taken to prevent job stress.

  ➢ *The Changing Organization of Work*—NORA Report

    This report was compiled as the first attempt in the United States to develop a comprehensive research agenda to investigate and reduce occupational safety and health risks associated with the changing organization of work. Four areas of research and development are targeted in the agenda.

  ➢ *Stress Management in Work Settings*—booklet

    This publication summarizes the scientific evidence and reviews conceptual and practical issues relating to worksite stress management. It is a collection of original contributions that address current issues and problems in the field.

> *Worker Health Chartbook 2004: Anxiety, Stress and Neurotic Disorders*—book (DHHS/NIOSH Publication No. 2004-146, 2004).

Provides data for anxiety and stress disorders based on magnitude and trend, age, sex, race/ethnicity, occupation, and industry.

12.15 National Institute of Mental Health (NIMH)

http://www.nimh.nih.gov

The NIMH is one of 27 components of the National Institutes of Health (NIMH), the federal government's principal biomedical and behavioral research agency concerned with the mental health of the nation. NIMH is part of the U.S. Department of Health and Human Services.

NIMH mental health information is based on scientific research and evidence-based practice. This information is compiled by NIMH to assist all those suffering from the problems of every day living, stress, and mental illnesses/disorders.

There appears to be as many responses to stress as there are people affected. Most individuals have intense feelings after a stressful traumatic event but completely recover. Others are more vulnerable—especially those who have had previous traumatic experiences—and need additional help.

Searching "stress" via the NIMH site provides click-on sites/reports including:
- *Reliving trauma: post-traumatic stress disorder*
- *Panic disorder: a real illness*
- *Mental health consequences of violence and disasters*
- *Center for the Study of Traumatic Stress—fact sheets*
- *Center for Disease Control (CDC)—fact sheet on Coping with Traumatic Events*

- *Men and depression: screening and treatment in primary care settings*
- *NIMH depression page: a resource area*
- *Depression and other serious illnesses*
- *Mental illnesses/disorders*

12.16 National Mental Health Association (NMHA)

http://www.nmha.org

NMHA is the USA's oldest and largest nonprofit organization addressing mental health and mental illness. With more than 340 affiliates nationwide, NMHA works to improve the mental health of all Americans, especially the 54 million people with mental disorders, through advocacy, education research and service.

Searching "stress" via the NMHA search site provides a number of click-on sites/reports concerning stress including:

- *Coping with Stress Checklist*
  http://nmha.org/infoctr/factsheets/stress.pdf
- *A Guide to Surviving Stress*
  http://www.nmha.org/mpower/411PopTopStress.htm
- *What is Mental Health*
  http://www.nmha.org/mpower/411PopTopMH.htm
- *Coming Home: How to Get Back to Normal*
  http://www.nmha.org/reassurance/cominghome/backtonormal.cfm
- *Coping with Disaster*
  http://www.nmha.org/reassurance/adulttips.cfm
- *Living Your Life During Terrorist Threats and Other Challenging Times*
  http://www.nmha.org/reassurance/terrorism.cfm

12.17 WebMD

http://www.webmd.com

WebMD is dedicated to providing quality health information and to upholding the integrity of their editorial policy—that health information provided is timely and credible. This website is reported to blend award winning expertise in medicine, journalism, health communication, and content creation to bring you the best health information possible. Their Medical Editorial Board and Independent Medical Review Board continuously reviews the site for accuracy and timeliness. MedicineNet.com makes frequent contributions to WebMD and comprises their Medical Editorial Board.

Searching "stress" and "stress management" on the WebMD website, a number of click-on sites are provided. Included are:

- *Effects of Stress*

  Stress can affect you both immediately (acute stress) and over time (chronic stress).

- *Avoiding Unnecessary Stress*

  Because stress is largely unavoidable in life, it is important to find ways to decrease and prevent stressful events.

- *Workplace Stress and Your Health*

  Experts explain the dangers of work-related stress and provide solutions.

- *Getting Out from Under Stress*

  Too much stress can cause physical and emotional problems.

- *Stress-free Stress Management*

  Does the thought of managing your stress cause you even more stress?

- *Stress Management Curbs Heart Disease*

  Exercise and stress management along with standard medical care may help the hearts of people.

- *Relieving Stress*

  Some of the most useful stress management skills you can learn are healthy coping strategies.

- *Dean Ornish's Life Style Components: Stress Management*

  Dean Ornish, MD's Lifestyle Program consists of four components: exercise, nutrition, stress management and a low stress healthy lifestyle.

- *Emotional Health—Coping with Stress, Depression and Anxiety*

  Get information on emotional health and wellness, plus advice to help you feeling your best.

Chapter 13—About the Author

Dr. DeFelice was born, raised and has lived all his life as a Roman Catholic.

His calling and purpose in life was to pursue a medical career of service based on a deep-seated desire to make the world a better place and serve mankind in a useful way. This calling and decision came about around age 14 following his mother's death in a diabetic coma, following witnessing her brother's death from burns and smoke inhalation after he rescued several fire victims while serving as a volunteer fireman.

After graduating from high school, the author enlisted and served in the U.S. Army of Occupation of Japan. Subsequently, he worked his way through Columbia University in New York City (B.S., 1951) and Boston University School of Medicine (M.D., 1956) and pursued a career in medicine and medical research.

Persistently and diligently building on his basic purpose in life, the author was able to develop the character, self-esteem, and inner strength (resilience) to endure and cope with the many hardships and stresses encountered to achieve a level of satisfaction and happiness in life for a "job well done"—making numerous contributions to medicine and medical research and helping many people along the way.

The Author's overall philosophy in life* is summarized in the short paragraph below.

---

* published as part of the Author's biographical sketch in Marquis' Who's Who in America

"Success in life comes from constancy of purpose, diligent work, living accord-ing to sound moral and religious principles, and having faith and hope in the future. Helping to make the world a better place to live in, autographing one's work in excellence, and doing good by others are the reward which brings happiness."

Eugene A. DeFelice, M.D., F.A.P.M. is an internationally recognized author, educator and retired Distinguished Clinical Professor of Medicine, UMDNJ-Robert Wood Johnson Medical School (1977–2003) and is listed in four separate Marquis reference publications, namely:

- Who's Who in America,
- Who's Who in American Education,
- Who's Who in Medicine and Healthcare, and
- Who's Who in the World

Also, the Author is a recipient of the Golden Merit Award of the Medical Society of New Jersey, having completed "Fifty Years of Distinguished Service as a Physician".

He is a Fellow of the Academy of Psychosomatic Medicine (F.A.P.M.) and the American Geriatric Society (A.G.S.F.), and author of over 70 med-ical/scientific articles and 12 books on medicine, nutrition, health and Web health resources. Books published include:

1. Stress and Health, iUniverse, Inc., 2006
2. Prevention of Cardiovascular Disease, iUniverse Inc., 2005
3. Web Health Information Resources, Second Edition, iUniverse Inc., 2004
4. Nutrition and Health, iUniverse, Inc. 2003
5. Overweight, Obesity and Health, iUniverse Inc., 2002
6. Breast Cancer, iUniverse Inc., 2002
7. Web Health Information Resource Guide, iUniverse, 2001

8. Angiotension Converting Enzyme Inhibitors, Alan R. Liss, 1987

9. Pharmacologic Treatment of Cardiovascular Disease, Elsevier, 1986

10. Beta Blockers in the Treatment of Cardiovascular Disease, Raven Press, 1984

11. Health and Obesity, Raven Press, 1983

12. Prostaglandins, Platelets, Lipids: New Developments in Atherosclerosis, Elsevier, 1981

978-0-595-41065-1
0-595-41065-0